The 90/10 Weight Loss Cookbook

Also by Joy Bauer
    The 90/10 Weight-Loss Plan
    The Complete Idiot's Guide to Total Nutrition

Also by Rosemary Black
    The Kids' Holiday Baking Book

The 90/10 Weight Loss Cookbook

Joy Bauer, M.S., R.D., C.D.N.

with Rosemary Black

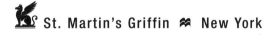 St. Martin's Griffin 🞄 New York

www.stmartins.com

Design by Leah Carlson-Stanisic

Library of Congress Caaloging-in-Publication Data

Bauer, Joy.
    The 90/10 weight loss cookbook / Joy Bauer, with Rosemary Black.
        p. cm.
    ISBN 0-312-31253-9 (hc)
    ISBN 0-312-33602-0 (pbk)
    EAN 978-0312-33602-8
    1. Low-calorie diet—Recipes I. Black, Rosemary. II. Title.

RM222.2.B38585 2004
613.2'5—dc22

                                        2003066805

First Published in the United States under the title *Cooking with Joy* by St. Martin's Press

First St. Martin's Griffin Edition: February 2005

10   9   8   7   6   5   4   3   2   1

For my wonderful parents, Ellen and Artie Schloss.
You empower me with confidence and love.

Contents

Acknowledgments

Many exceptional people were involved in the creation of this book, including colleagues who helped with fact-finding and recipe development, friends and family who lent their taste buds (over and over again), publishing professionals who put the entire puzzle together, and my extraordinary clients who constantly remind me what works, and what doesn't. I am eternally grateful to all of them.

First, let me personally thank Rosemary Black—it's an honor to have your name on my book. You're a fabulous writer, cook, superstar mom, and special friend. You have my deepest respect and gratitude . . . and six kids! Unbelievable.

A tremendous thanks to my literary agent, Jane Dystel. You're always there to guide me in the right direction and I appreciate every minute of it.

To my wonderful editor, Heather Jackson, whose ingenious capabilities helped to transform *Cooking with Joy* into a full-blown kitchen bible. I feel lucky to have had the opportunity to work with you.

To the entire crew at St. Martin's Press, your enthusiasm and dedication are greatly appreciated. Special thanks to Sally Richardson and Matthew Shear for giving me this opportunity, Mike Storrings for making my books sparkle, Elizabeth Bewley for all that you do, John Murphy and Yamil Anglada for publicity, and Elizabeth Catalano for her production expertise.

To Kyle Shadix, M.S., R.D., a talented chef, expert nutritionist, and one hell of a great guy! Thanks for providing your dynamite recipes. They're scrumptious.

To Veronica Laslo for sharing your Chicken Paprika, and to Rebecca Gainen for your secret cookie potion. Also, big thanks to Hiranth Jayasinghe and Brett Ludy at BlueEarth Caterers in New York City, for lending two fabulous recipes.

To my unstoppable research team: Polina, M.S., R.D., Mili Desai, M.S., R.D., Alyse Levine, M.S.,

R.D.E., and Rebecca Gainen, M.S., R.D.E. Appreciation is an understatement! Thanks to your diligence and attention to detail, we covered it all.

A special thanks to the folks who shared their 90/10 success stories: L.W., Harold I., Laura C., and Sara M.

To my guinea-pig taste testers: The Beal family: Debra, Steve, Ben, Noah, Harvey, and Jenny (Becca, I'll get you on the next book). The Schloss family: Ellen, Artie, Pam, Dan, Charlie, and Glenn. The Bauer family: Carol, Vic, Jason, Harley, and Mia. The Malachowsky family: Mary and Nat. The Farruggio family: Nancy, Sal, Brielle, and Andrew. The Cohen/Shapiro family: Nancy, Jon, and Camrin. And a special thanks to Lisi Epstein, Shannon Green, Maria Santoro, and many others who had no idea what they were in for when they entered my house.

To ABC's *Good Morning America* producers Patty Neger and Janice Johnston for giving me the opportunity to serve my recipes at our "Lock the Door, Lose the Weight" segment series.

To John Ottavino for making me feel glamorous. And, of course, special thanks to Cindy Cinicolo and Louisa Guigli.

To the dedicated dietitians/nutritionists at Joy Bauer Nutrition: Lisa Mandelbaum, Jennifer Medina, Maria Baldo, Elyssa Hurlbut, Laura Pumillo, Erica Ilton, Nicole DiLorenzo, Suzanne Magnotta, Lisa Young, Betty Kovacs, and Katherine Brooking. Thanks for your advice, opinions, and energy.

Most important, I'd like to thank my family for making my life shine: my husband, Ian, and my three children, Jesse, Cole, and Ayden Jane. I just love you so much!

Introduction

Stuck in a diet rut? Convinced that you'll be on the gain-and-lose seesaw for life? Think you'll never look the way you want to look? You're wrong. This unique book will revolutionize the way you think about food and how you prepare it. *Cooking with Joy* is the follow-up to my best-selling *90/10 Weight-Loss Plan.* My first book walks you through a detailed diet regimen. It's based on the realistic food strategy: eat healthy 90 percent of the time and have fun the other 10 percent. This new book further educates you about how to lose weight, maintain a healthy lifestyle, and become savvy in your kitchen without feeling hungry or deprived.

This book enhances your 90/10 success by educating you on shopping smart, helping you to become comfortable with cooking, and providing more than one hundred new recipes that are perfectly calculated to fit into my original 90/10 weight-loss regimen. Even if you are *not* trying to shed pounds or not following my original *90/10 Weight-Loss Plan, Cooking with Joy* offers valuable information that will be beneficial to your health and overall well-being.

You'll learn how to decipher a nutrition label, how to decide which meats and poultry are worth buying, and how to zero in on the finest, freshest fruits and vegetables. I explain the best method for shopping for everything from breads to cereals to dairy products with an eye toward getting the best nutritional buys. And I steer you away from the high-fat, high-sugar foods that are sure to undermine your weight-loss regimen. I even provide you with the best bets in brand-name items.

What's more, this is a book for everyone to cook from: those who are into fitness and those who are totally clueless about nutrition, people of every weight and body type, and those from every economic background. As mentioned earlier, it's got an information-packed shopping chapter that will make you feel like a supermarket expert. And my cooking strategies will have you expertly preparing low-fat braised meats, sautéed vegetables, and delicious stir-fries that taste so good you won't want to follow them up with empty-calorie, high-fat snacks.

If you've followed my *90/10 Weight-Loss Plan,* you know how it works. Aimed at helping you experience fast, effective, and healthy weight loss, it includes ample amounts of nutritious fare, coupled with portion-controlled fun indulgences. It's a plan that makes you feel motivated and satisfied, and it's easy to follow, since all the 90/10 menus are carefully calculated to maximize nutritional intake while keeping total calories low enough to guarantee weight loss.

My entire food strategy is based on 90 percent healthy and 10 percent fun. Roughly 90 percent of your food intake should come from healthful, well-balanced meals, while 10 percent is the average amount of calories that should come from fun food choices. Of course, it's not an exact math; in fact the percentages range from 80 percent healthy and 20 percent fun to 100 percent healthy and 0 percent fun—depending on what plan you're following and which fun food you choose on a given day.

That said, 90/10 is a food philosophy that works not just for quick weight loss but, even better, for long-term weight management. I'm a firm believer that folks should lose weight eating the very same foods that they'll be eating after the weight is lost. And let's face it—we love to eat non-dietetic foods! My *90/10 Weight-Loss Plan* teaches life-long eating for health—a smart, sane food plan that you really can use for the rest of your life.

The reason I know it will work for you is that I've seen it work over and over again. In my nutrition practice I have met thousands of unsuccessful dieters who failed because they tried losing weight with an eating plan that was unpleasantly different from the way they normally ate. My plan differs because it's reasonable, easy to follow, and effortless to maintain.

In my original book, I presented three separate caloric plans for those trying to lose weight: 1,200, 1,400, and 1,600. In this book, I have included caloric breakdowns for two additional meal plans: an 1,800-calorie and a 2,000-calorie regimen tailored to active people, nearly all men, and those who have already lost the weight and now are determined to keep those pounds off. If you want to jump right in and incorporate these recipes into a complete weight-loss plan, I also present a rotation diet for both meat eaters and vegetarians. And for 90/10 participants, I break down the recipes into portion sizes *and* side accompaniments for every plan: 1,200; 1,400; 1,600; 1,800; and 2,000 calories a day. The math is done, so you can simply enjoy cooking and eating delicious meals tailored to your personal weight management goal. What's more, a complete nutritional analysis follows every recipe. So for 90/10 participants and for folks who simply want to know more about the foods they eat, I list how many calories and how much protein, carbohydrates, sugar, fat, saturated fat, cholesterol, sodium, fiber, and calcium are in each dish. Say you have osteoporosis and you are trying to boost your intake of calcium, and maybe you also are determined to lower your LDL cholesterol numbers. You can scout out the dishes that are high in calcium and low in dietary cholesterol and saturated fat. And if you have high blood pressure and/or irritable bowel syndrome, you can select recipes that are lower in sodium and higher in fiber.

My 90/10 plan isn't only for you, it's also for your family. Say good-bye to those harried nights of cooking one meal for your spouse and children and something entirely different for you. Now you can all enjoy the same meals (yours, of course, are portion-controlled and supplemented by plenty of nutrient-packed raw and cooked vegetables).

This book is full of information to help you rethink how you feel about food and your body, teach you how to keep the weight off, and how you can maintain good health while feeling perfectly satisfied with the foods you eat.

Part I offers a wealth of information on preparing your 90/10 kitchen. In "Shopping Smart," I transform you into an expert consumer at your local grocery store—purchasing the best nutritional bets in everything from yogurt to eggs, beef, whole grains, and marinades. I explain the difference between "90 percent fat-free" and "95 percent lean" on the label of a package of ground turkey and give you name-brand recommendations for the best cold cuts, frozen dinners, bacon, hot dogs, and vegetarian options. Also in this chapter is a Nutrition Label Cheat Sheet, which provides definitions for everything from "low-calorie" and "reduced-fat" to "cholesterol-free" and "low-sodium," so you can tell at a glance what these terms mean and how a particular food fits into your meal plan. I even give you the details on the most recent organic labeling laws.

In "Cooking ABC's," every aspect of kitchen management is covered in detail, from how to store foods you buy to how to turn a humble vegetable or inexpensive piece of meat into a delectable meal. Whether you are trying to lose weight, maintain your goal weight, or simply ensure that you and your family are following a well-balanced, healthy eating plan, this chapter is a must-read. It contains useful information and how-to techniques guaranteed to make you a savvier cook as you learn to steam, stir-fry, and sauté with a bare minimum of oil.

I give quick ideas for perfect meats and vegetables, tell you how to oven-roast vegetables until they are super-sweet, crisp outside and soft inside—so good you'd happily choose these over greasy potato chips any day. Here's where you learn how to boost the flavor of foods with ingredients that add little in the way of fat or calories—a sprinkling of fresh herbs under the skin of a chicken to infuse the meat with delicious flavor, and a tablespoon of toasted nuts to add color and crunch to a salad. Garnishing and dressing up plates of foods like the pros do can go a long way toward making each and every meal look as special as it tastes, and most of these little tricks and tips can be accomplished in minutes, with very little effort. This chapter also has useful information on measurements, substitutions, and equivalents, so the next time you need to know how many cups a pound of broccoli equals, or what you can substitute when you have no tomato paste, you'll be able to find the answer.

Part II presents more than one hundred recipes to excite your taste buds and impress guests. There are recipes for breakfast, lunch, dinner, and dessert which satisfy every craving and holiday occasion. My recipe collection covers the gamut, from simple fare for weekdays to gourmet meals to serve guests and enjoy with your family on holidays. There are breakfasts, lunches, and dinners here, along with a tremendous variety of both sweet and savory fun food recipes. Breakfasts range from a low-fat granola that you can eat on the run to mouthwatering scones packed with fresh cranberries and pecans—the perfect breakfast to savor on a weekend.

If you are trying to pump good-tasting protein into your lunches, I offer Egg White Vegetable Dijonnaise, Cape Cod Tuna Salad, and Three-Cheese Quesadillas. Vegetarians can feast on Cool Tabbouleh with Mint and Black Bean and Spinach Burritos.

The dinner chapter truly has something for everyone. If you're a beef lover, you'll enjoy my Herb-Marinated Flank Steak and Slow-Cooker Beef Stroganoff, while seafood fans can enjoy Shrimp with Garlic and Feta, Asian Citrus Salmon Steak, and Lemon Pepper–Seared Tuna Steaks. And if you're looking for poultry, enjoy scrumptious recipes such as Chicken Mushroom Marinara, Chicken Dijon, and Tex-Mex Turkey Burgers.

"Kids in the Kitchen" includes all the recipes that your children will enjoy preparing and gobbling down: Tacos, Peanut Butter and Jelly Rolls, Trail Mix, and Pretty in Pink Strawberry Soup will help to start them on a lifetime of healthy eating. There's plenty of advice on how to encourage your children to maintain good eating habits as well as tips on how to make family dinnertime pleasurable and relaxing. Incorporating 90/10 strategies into your kids' meals teaches them to love nutritious, healthful dishes, along with fun foods that are as fun to make as they are to eat. And although the regular 90/10 recipes are all terrific for kids as well as adults, I include a batch of kid-tested, kid-friendly recipes. Try Cucumber Tuna Ship, Rainbow Chicken Nuggets, and Frankie and His Friends, for starters! And, finally, there's the incredible fun foods chapter! Here are Oreo Vanilla Pudding Pie, Strawberry-Topped Cheesecake, and Angel Food Cake with Fresh Berries. If you crave snacks that are savory, try Hot Artichoke Dip and Oven-Baked French Fries.

I created most of these recipes with Rosemary Black, and we double-tested every one on our toughest critics (our husbands and children) as well as on friends. The recipes in "Gourmet Dinners and Festive Holiday Menus" were developed by Kyle Shadix, M.S., R.D., a talented chef and nutritionist with a real flair for combining flavors in a creative way.

Cooking with Joy is a collection of expert advice on every aspect of food selection and preparation. It's filled with creative and delicious recipes for every meal of the day and is a book you'll cook from again and again. Enjoy reading the following pages. They will show you how to lose weight, maintain good health, and look wonderful. Bon appetit!

Part I Preparing Your 90/10 Kitchen

One

90/10 Success!

As you know all too well if you've tried one diet after another in your quest to lose weight—from a pill-popping regimen to a protein-to-carb ratio—there is no magic formula for effortlessly shedding unwanted pounds. The only genuine, time-tested principle of healthy, long-term weight loss is to take in fewer calories than your body burns. That said, the best way to sustain a calorie-controlled diet is through portion control and cravings satisfaction. These must be perfectly balanced in order for a plan to be successful—portion control doesn't work in the long run if you constantly feel hungry and deprived.

To come up with a plan that would guarantee weight-loss success without that starved, weak feeling that frequently goes hand in hand with a "restrictive" diet, I created a weight-reduction regimen that would meet my clients' health needs while simultaneously satisfying their appetites. This is also a highly workable, satisfying plan to follow even if you don't need to lose weight. All of us, whether or not we want to lose weight, should take pride in what we put into our bodies. And if you are trying to coax your family into eating more healthfully, this may be just the inspiration you need to start cooking nutritious, delectable meals your partner and your children will love.

An Overview of the 90/10 Weight-Loss Plan

My original book, *The 90/10 Weight-Loss Plan*, was written for those who want to lose weight. The book presented three solid meal plans that promote fast, effective, long-term weight loss. Each plan was calculated to include all types of food in a healthy balance so you wind up feeling satisfied—and motivated to stick with it.

Many trendy fad diets focus on omitting entire food groups or on simply counting fat and/or carbohydrate grams. But 90/10 is a scientifically designed, flexible plan that allows for a substantial amount of personal choice. Each daily menu is calculated to provide generous amounts of nutrition, while still keeping the total calories low enough so that you will lose weight. Here's where my fun foods come in. About 10 percent of the calories in a typical day come from fun food choices, though the ratio can vary. In fact, it can vary from 0 to 20 percent, depending on which plan you follow and which fun foods you choose or don't choose to plug in. Fun foods are all portion controlled at 250 calories or fewer and include favorites such as chocolate, ice cream, potatoes, cookies, and more. Furthermore, each day I give the option of forgoing the fun food and instead adding 250 calories of healthier options. The choice is yours. You'll also note that some fun foods offer not just fun but nutrition as well. Frozen yogurt, cheese, nuts, and peanut butter are some of these foods that offer a double bonus. In this new book, packed with all types of delicious recipes, I also present healthier fun food options that offer nutrition along with indulgence—for example, homemade guacamole, a good source of monounsaturated fat as well as beta-carotene, and low-fat, low-sugar chocolate mousse, packed with calcium.

My food philosophy doesn't focus on exact math; instead it promotes an overall weight-loss strategy. It's a realistic food plan, one that works beautifully because it concentrates on the behavioral changes that are so important for permanent weight loss—changes that will indeed transform your life. Thanks to a balance of the foods you crave and the foods you need to be healthy and feel good, followers of the 90/10 plan feel satisfied both physically and emotionally. No matter what your dieting history, you'll soon discover that this is a plan you can commit to for life. The original meal plan (now with the recipes in this book) enables you to get all the nutrients your body needs and is designed to provide you with the most vitamins and minerals possible for the controlled amount of calories consumed.

The menus in *The 90/10 Weight-Loss Plan* are low in dietary cholesterol and saturated fat, and high in fiber, antioxidants, and phytochemicals, all of which can help reduce your risk of heart disease and some cancers, promote healthy digestion, and improve circulation. Of course, the recipes in *Cooking with Joy* all follow suit. Once you start to follow the 90/10 plan, you'll most likely feel more positive and energetic. That's because you're feeding your body with the right mix of food, and you're in complete control. No more bouncing from restrictive plans to bingeing on "forbidden" foods. All the foods you need and crave are part of the program.

With the recipes in this book, I've done all the calorie crunching, so that every recipe is presented in portion-controlled servings. What's more, all the breakfast portions within a specific plan are calorie-equivalent, as are the lunches, dinners, and snacks. Thus, you never have to eat anything you don't like and you can certainly repeat recipes as often as you like. These recipes are all interchangeable with the menus and recipes in the fourteen-day meal plan outlined in my original book, as well as any other calorie-controlled plan you may be following. They are all healthy, delicious, and satisfying dishes to add to your repertoire of mealtime fare.

Because success is based on maximizing nutrition and controlling calories, you need to know the right amount of calories for your personal weight-loss goals. If you've followed my plan in the past, you're set. For newcomers, determine your appropriate caloric level by considering the following criteria.

How Many Calories Do You Need?

The fewest amount of calories recommended for good health is 1,200 per day. My 1,200-calorie plan is for women who either don't exercise or exercise two hours or fewer per week and don't work in a physically demanding job. Also, if you are postmenopausal and over age fifty, you might want to consider this plan as well. Short women, five foot two or less, with a small amount of weight to lose should also consider starting on this plan.

My 1,400-calorie plan works well for *nearly all* women. Consider this one if you have a moderately active lifestyle, if you are between the ages of eighteen and fifty, and/or if you have from two to fifty pounds to lose. The 1,600-calorie plan works well for nearly all men, although it may not be enough food for men taller than five foot six. Women above five foot six may also choose this plan, as taller people automatically have additional lean body mass and thus a higher baseline metabolism (more calories to play with). Even if you are shorter, if you are a diligent exerciser who works out at least five times per week, you may want to follow this plan, as it will help to fuel and optimize your vigorous workouts. My 1,800-calorie plan is for active men, and my 2,000-calorie plan is for tall men who are very active, as well as for other 90/10 followers who've already lost the weight and are determined to keep the pounds off but want a more liberal eating plan.

No matter which plan you opt to follow, remember that the 90/10 philosophy is not written in stone! Obviously, there will be days when you will go off your plan completely, either at a meal or at snacktime. My advice is: Don't give up on the entire day! Just count the excessive food as a "meal *plus* your fun food." Then carry on with healthful food choices. In fact, throw in some extra exercise to rid yourself of those extra calories and clear your head of any guilt or remorse.

What if you feel hungry or hypoglycemic while following the 90/10 plan? Certainly you can spread out your meals or add an extra snack when your body requires it. A small additional snack should not impede your weight-loss effort. Suggestions for reasonably sized snacks include a serving of fruit or a vegetable, a nonfat yogurt, or a slice of reduced-calorie whole wheat bread with a teaspoon of peanut butter or a slice of low-fat cheese. If you consistently feel hungry and lightheaded, you may need to be eating more. Some people start at one calorie level and move to another, depending on their weight loss and hunger. Remember, this is not a race. It's a lifelong way of eating.

Often it can be helpful to know the exact calorie breakdown for each plan, so check out the box below that presents the math for each of the five plans. This can help when certain foods are not available or practical. For example, say you are in a situation where you can't cook a 90/10 meal from scratch and your only alternative is a frozen entrée from the supermarket. This is perfectly okay, provided that the substituted meal falls within the correct caloric range. So long as you stay within these caloric guidelines, you may alter a few 90/10 meals to fit your personal tastes. Of course try to keep these substitutions to a minimum. I designed these menus to provide well-balanced nutrition, and to replace nutritious meals with less-than-healthy alternatives is counter-productive.

Calorie Breakdowns for 90/10 Weight Loss Plan

1,200-CALORIE PLAN

Breakfast: 200 calories
Lunch: 300 calories
Snack: 100 calories
Dinner: 350 calories
Fun food: 250 calories (or fewer)

1,400-CALORIE PLAN

Breakfast: 250 calories
Lunch: 350 calories
Snack: 100 calories
Dinner: 450 calories
Fun food: 250 calories (or fewer)

1,600-CALORIE PLAN

Breakfast: 250 calories
Lunch: 400 calories
Snack: 150 calories
Dinner: 550 calories
Fun food: 250 calories (or fewer)

1,800-CALORIE PLAN

Breakfast: 300 calories
Lunch: 500 calories
Snack: 200 calories
Dinner: 550 calories
Fun food: 250 calories (or fewer)

2,000-CALORIE PLAN

Breakfast: 350 calories
Lunch: 500 calories
Snack: 250 calories
Dinner: 650 calories
Fun food: 250 calories (or fewer)

Some Things to Keep in Mind

BEVERAGES

You may drink unlimited plain coffee or tea throughout the day, but if you are caffeine-sensitive, limit your consumption. (If you're taking medication or have a preexisting medical condition, ask your doctor what caffeine allowance is suitable for you.) You may substitute low-fat soy milk and/or Lactaid milk for skim milk on any of the 90/10 food plans. You may also enjoy as much water and noncaloric seltzer as you like. Try no-calorie flavored varieties of seltzer, or squeeze in your own fresh lemon. If you enjoy chewing gum, you may have one standard pack per day of any sugarless chewing gum you like. Just the act of chewing can be enough to keep you from eating high-calorie foods.

SIDES

Each dinner recipe has a suggested "side" of a salad, vegetable, or both. All vegetables listed with any dinner may be substituted with any of the following vegetables on a given night (the portion size stays the same): asparagus, beets, broccoli, Brussels sprouts, cabbage, carrots, cauliflower, celery, cucumbers, eggplant, green beans, greens (collard, mustard, and turnip), kohlrabi, leeks, lettuce, mushrooms, okra, onions, pea pods, peppers (red, yellow, and green), radishes, rutabaga, spinach, tomatoes, water chestnuts, and zucchini. And if you're feeling extra hungry, you can always increase these vegetable servings on any given day.

SPICING THINGS UP

Whenever you feel like spicing up a dish with herbs and other seasonings, you may use unlimited amounts of any of the following: basil, bay leaves, celery seeds, chervil, chili powder, chives, cinnamon, cumin, curry, dill, flavoring extracts (such as almond, vanilla, and walnut), garlic powder, hot pepper sauce, lemon juice, lemon pepper, lime juice, minced onion or onion powder, oregano, paprika, parsley, pepper, pimiento, rosemary, sage, low-sodium soy sauce, tarragon, thyme, turmeric, and vinegar.

MEATLESS MEALS

Vegetarians may substitute tofu or tempeh for appropriate recipes that include meat, chicken, or fish. When substituting tofu, just double the ounces listed for meat, chicken, or fish. For tempeh, the ounces remain the same as those listed for meat, fish, or chicken. Soy cheese or vegetable cheese may be substituted for regular low-fat/nonfat cheese, and low-fat soy milk may be substituted for skim milk (the amounts remain the same).

Above all, keep in mind that the 90/10 strategy is designed to help you feel good about your ability to control and choose your food while at the same time allowing you to indulge in those daily fun foods. This plan dares to acknowledge that we love cake, cookies, rich desserts, and starchy carbs. Therefore, I have portion-controlled these favorite indulgences right into the plan. All foods can now work for you. And keep in mind that once you've reached your weight-loss goal, you can effortlessly incorporate the 90/10 plan into your life. Enjoy eating a whole lot of healthy foods . . . mixed with a bit of fun.

Now that you understand the 90/10 philosophy, *Cooking with Joy* offers a tremendous bonus for both dieters and folks who want to maintain good health with great tasting food. In the following chapters, I'll provide you with the ultimate guide for shopping smart and present step-by-step cooking techniques that will help you prepare sensational low-calorie meals on a daily basis. But, before we begin, enjoy reading a few 90/10 success stories. They are quite inspirational!

90/10 Success!

I'd like to thank the following 90/10 participants for sharing their motivating stories. Use their success to help you get started and for constant inspiration. I'm sure you'll find a few similarities in their journey, which may move you toward a healthier relationship with food and help you achieve long-term weight management.

Sara didn't have a weight problem until she entered middle school. Before that she was so active that she could eat whatever she wanted and not gain excess weight. But once she got into the sixth grade and the homework piled up, the pounds piled on. She spent a lot of time studying and grew more sedentary with each year. High school was even worse—Sara just kept gaining weight, until by graduation day she was so ashamed of the way she looked that she didn't even want to dress up in a cap and gown. Although she loved eating just about anything, her real weakness was chocolate bars and anything salty.

Sara tried numerous weight-loss regimens. But every diet she tried ended in dismal failure. After seeing commercials for various pills and potions that promised magically to melt off the pounds, she'd try yet another plan. She wanted a quick fix, but those stubborn pounds refused to budge.

At just five feet tall, Sara has a small frame, and soon after she entered college, she ballooned up to 180 pounds. Besides feeling desperate about her appearance, Sara hated that she didn't have any energy at all. It took her forever to climb up three flights of stairs to some of her classes. She finally began to take the service elevator just so she wouldn't arrive winded, flustered, and sweaty. But there was a big sign on the elevator: "Unless you are in a wheelchair or carrying something very heavy, you're not permitted to ride on this." Of course, whenever she got off the elevator and there were people around, she was embarrassed.

Around Christmastime, Sara happened to see me talking on a local Tulsa TV program about my 90/10 program. A few months went by before she started the plan herself. By the end of the summer, after six months on the plan, she had lost sixty pounds.

Sara found that following the 90/10 plan was practically effortless. The key to her willpower was knowing that at the end of the day, she could still unwind and enjoy a fun food—her chocolate bar fix! Like so many 90/10 followers, she quickly figured out how to make this plan work for her. For Sara, that meant saving the fun food for later in the night. She never felt deprived. The days turned into weeks, which turned into months, and before she knew it, she was feeling great, looking great, and destined never to be overweight again.

At the same time, Sara began exercising. A history buff who loves to read, write, and surf the Internet, her lifestyle tends to be sedentary. Although she can't run because she has trouble with her knees, she took up walking. Before long, Sara was doing five or six miles each night. In addition to helping her lose weight, that sixty to ninety minutes of walking five days a week did wonders for her stress level and muscle tone! She now feels better both physically and mentally.

Now that she has lost the weight, Sara has been very successful in sticking to a maintenance plan. Although she started out on the 1,200-calorie plan, she now eats between 1,400 and 1,800 calories per day. Recently accepted into law school, she's looking forward with confidence to lifting heavy books, putting in sixteen-hour days—and running up the stairs to her classes instead of sneaking off to take the freight elevator!

Douglas, fifty-three years old, is five foot eight and weighed more than 300 pounds. He'd been a big-time high school and college football player who got on the spiral of gaining and gaining. Suffering from high blood sugar and cholesterol, along with elevated triglycerides, he was on medication for hypertension. Because of his high blood pressure and type 2 diabetes, his doctor (and his wife, who is a nurse) urged him to lose weight. A senior executive with a big consulting company, Douglas is constantly traveling. As a "road warrior" who lives on airplanes, in hotel rooms, and in conference rooms, he has no time whatsoever for himself, but he made time to see me.

After our initial consultation I genuinely felt he'd be a tremendous success. We created a meal plan around airplanes, traveling, and long days and nights; we became a dynamic team. Because Douglas had so much excess weight, he lost 10 pounds in the first two weeks. A month later, he was down 20 pounds. By the end of the next month, he'd shed 28 pounds, his blood glucose was normal, and his cholesterol level was under 200.

Five months later, Douglas had lost 70 pounds. He is aiming to get down to 200 pounds, and I have no doubt that he will accomplish this, too. Often at night, for his fun food, he has a mug of

90/10 Recovery

Written by an extraordinary client who conquered a battle of disordered eating.

I've learned a valuable lesson over the years. Weight is not as uncontrollable as many of us think it is. I've been on both extremes of the scale: I've been referred to as "big boned" and "solid" any number of times, and I've also been called "skinny Minnie" and "lollipop."

In grammar school, while my friends were joining Girl Scout troops, I was happy to stay home and financially support bake sales by eating. I was lively and opinionated, but I didn't understand deeper emotions. Instead, I ate.

In high school, I never lost my desire for thinness, but I did falter many a time in my active pursuit of it. Southern California is well stocked with the kind of long-legged blondes who will give any ordinary person a complex. It wasn't long before I'd developed as solid a relationship with my toilet bowl as I had with the kitchen pantry. Bulimia seems like a great idea to most overeaters, but the truth is that it does little more than destroy your internal organs. For the most part, I reached a point where I could control it, but the overeating never stopped.

By the time I reached college, I'd come to see myself as a failure-riddled second-class citizen who didn't have much to offer the world. I spent most of my days at Barnes & Noble, huddled over a scone with my head in a book. Of course, I spent all kinds of time pitying myself that I couldn't get a date, but it never occurred to me that it had anything to do with never talking to anyone. I was stuck in a terrible cycle: assuming that being overweight made me less attractive, then acting less attractive, which simply made me what I imagined, and I felt bad because I was treated accordingly. Weight is such an easy defense, no matter what the game.

The summer after freshman year of college, I worked at a restaurant. Every day I showed up for work with my knees shaking, and every night when I got into my car I burst into tears of relief. When I finally gathered up the courage to give my two-week notice after a month of complete turmoil, I was forced to admit utter defeat. I was an official failure; I couldn't even survive the most basic of jobs. Then something inside me clicked, and I decided that I was going to take control of my life.

Over the next two years, I changed just about everything in my life. I went from a C average to a 4.0 GPA, got a great internship at a major magazine, and lost more than 60 pounds. I went from a size fourteen to a size zero in Gap jeans and still felt like a cow. At the same time, I developed a rather complex relationship with the outside world. I reveled in the inevitable compliments but resented what felt like reinforcement of my previous ugliness. Aside from the time I spent studying, I think it's safe to say that I never ever stopped thinking about food. It had become my best friend. I took long New York City walks and taunted myself, staring into the windows of bakeries and wandering the aisles of gourmet grocery stores. "Look at all that food I can't eat." I'd sit and read cookbooks at Barnes & Noble, constructing some imaginary feast at which I gorged on all the forbidden foods. Coconut rice! Olive oil focaccia! Apple pie! Gruyère fondue, chocolate layer cake, buttermilk biscuits, chocolate ganache!

Despite how seriously ill I was becoming as my anorexia persisted, it took a series of events for me to stop the starvation. It took an angry brother, a gossipy friend, and an assortment of physical side effects like bone loss and amenorrhea (lack of menstruation). It took professional help to really change my habits. It took time to establish non-emotional eating habits that were still psychologically rewarding. That was the most important thing—learning to eat in a way that acknowledged my body's needs for fuel and moderation but also my mind's need for satisfaction and pleasure.

Joy calls her plan a "90/10 food strategy." I call it "spinach and ice cream." By the same token, nothing was more beneficial than establishing a middle ground with my food.

I now take long walks, I drink a lot of water, and I eat food that's good for me. However, moments of spontaneity are equally important, and I try to keep life interesting with random dance classes, weekday movie matinees, Twizzlers, and other portion-controlled foods that used to be off-limits.

These days, I make it a point to be aware of my strengths and abilities. I'm a success at many things, and I don't need to prove myself through my eating habits anymore. Life is hard, food should be easy.

low-fat ice cream, and he typically plugs in extra fruit here and there during the day as needed. (Believe me, that bowl of ice cream and the extra fruit are nothing compared to the amount of carbs he used to consume!) Other times his fun food is automatically worked into his daily menu with unexpected "extras" at business meetings, client dinners, and visits to the late-night hospitality suite in his hotel.

By the fifth month on my plan, Douglas was motivated to begin a formal exercise regimen, which he has continued to maintain. He also walks to and from appointments much more than he ever did before, and he reports feeling much less winded when he takes the stairs (amazing achievement!). Douglas's long-term goal is to knock off another 50 pounds, feel and look better than he did in college, and start playing football again for fun with friends. Douglas brags that he is now able to zip up an old, favorite aviator jacket. He feels better than he has in a long time and loves seeing the transformation in himself. He is looking forward to getting off his blood pressure medication . . . and shopping for new clothes.

Now that you understand how real people have changed their lives with my 90/10 plan, you're ready to dive in and give your kitchen a makeover. The following chapter will show you how to make smart choices in the grocery store and how to navigate your way through the aisles with the best bets in low-fat dairy, grains, produce, meat, fish, poultry, and condiments.

Two

Shopping Smart

Let's face it. A lot of the eating we do is not when we're hungry, but when we're bored, procrastinating, anxious, or stressed over something. Of course, when the urge to nosh strikes and we head for the kitchen, we tend to grab whatever's in sight, no matter how high it is in fat, salt, and sugar. Over and over, we sabotage our own weight-loss success simply because we stock our cupboards and refrigerators with the wrong foods.

Before you even start planning and cooking healthful meals and snacks for you and your family, let's go on an aisle-by-aisle shopping excursion to the supermarket. The key to your weight-loss success is learning which products are the smartest buys for people trying to manage their weight, which aisles should definitely be off-limits, and where you'll find the freshest, healthiest foods to satisfy your hunger as well as those uncontrollable cravings.

Rule #1: Make a grocery list and take it with you to the store.

Going food shopping without a list is like setting off to an unfamiliar destination without a map. You're bound to get lost along the way, forget the things you came to buy, and wind up choosing all kinds of things you don't need or want. Rather than wandering aimlessly down every aisle, impulsively tossing whatever strikes your fancy into your cart, figure out in advance just what you'll be cooking for the coming week, and stick to these purchases.

To save money as well as time, carefully review the ads in your local newspapers and circulars to find out the week's specials. That way, when lean boneless loin of pork is on sale you can pick one up and prepare a family-pleasing entrée, like Apple Dijon–Encrusted Loin of Pork, in the gourmet dinner chapter.

Resolving to stick to your list also keeps you focused on what you should be eating. You know what your "problem" foods are; try to avoid the aisles containing them or, if you must go down that aisle, know in advance exactly what you need—and put your blinders on to everything else! In fact, the more you can stay out of the center aisles of the store, the better off you are. Shop the perimeter of the supermarket, which is where you'll find low-fat dairy products, fresh fruits and vegetables, and lean meat and seafood. Supermarkets know that it's hard to resist the temptations that beckon as you make your way from the front of the store to the back, so try as much as possible to steer clear of this aisle-by-aisle danger zone and stick with buying the basics at the edges of the store.

Rule #2: Never go shopping hungry.

Shopping on an empty stomach causes you to overbuy—and often overeat, when store employees are handing out free food items to tempt you. Say you're going to the supermarket on the way home from work. You're exhausted and so famished you'd eat anything, so you buy everything in sight. If, on the other hand, you have a small snack before heading off to the store, you're much more likely to resist temptation. Pop a piece of gum in your mouth and take a cup of coffee or tea or a bottle of water into the store with you. If the coffee or tea has a secure top on it, keep it in the cart and sip on it occasionally as you reach for items. It'll last you the whole trip, and that oral gratification will keep you from consuming those tempting, high-calorie impulse foods or busting open one of your own purchases (we've all done it!).

Rule #3: Try to leave the kids at home and go to the store by yourself.

For one thing, you'll be able to focus on reading nutrition labels without worrying that your toddler will fall out of a shopping cart or your preschooler will race down the aisle out of sight. For another, our darlings have a habit of pleading and begging for the very foods it's hard for you to pass up when your resistance is down. So shop solo, even if it means having to go in the evening when you can leave the kids at home with your mate.

Your Aisle-by-Aisle Guide

Plan to spend the majority of your shopping trip in the fresh produce section. Here, load your cart with nutrient-high, calorie-low fresh fruits and vegetables that fill you up and make you feel good. Try lots of different kinds of fruits and veggies in order to find ones you really like—these can be the solution to the problem of what to do when you have the urge to snack. They're crunchy, they take a long time to eat, and you can usually pack them by the baggie-full to take to work, on a long car ride, even to your child's field trip.

VEGETABLES

Vegetables are powerhouses of vitamins, minerals, soluble and insoluble fiber, as well as other phytonutrients. And except for olives and avocados, few produce items contain much in the way of fat or calories. (It's true the fat in olives and avocados boosts calories and perhaps impedes weight loss; however, it is important to note that the fat is monounsaturated, which may help prevent heart disease and promote overall wellness.)

Another exception to the carte blanche vegetable rule is to go easy with the amount and frequency of starchier vegetables. Although starchy vegetables provide ample nutrition, they unfortunately have more calories compared to non-starchy varieties. These starchier veggies include corn, peas, potatoes, lima beans, and butternut and acorn squash.

Be sure to examine all produce carefully and avoid any with bruises. And buy only what you can use for a few days, as many fresh fruits and veggies get overripe and unappetizing if they sit around in your fridge for a long time. If you can't shop often, buy frozen vegetables. They come cut, whole, chopped, and pureed, so there is very little prep time required. And since freezing locks in nutrients, you don't have to hurry to eat them before they spoil. Be sure to avoid frozen vegetable medleys that come in a sauce, as these can be high in fat and calories. Always read the label to make sure there isn't a lot of added salt and fat. Simply put, keep it plain. Many of our recipes call for either fresh or frozen vegetables, so it's your choice: Let your lifestyle dictate which route you go.

Vegetable	Amount per serving	Calories (kcal)	Fiber (g)	Rich In	Tips	Storage
Asparagus	5 spears	18	1.7	Potassium, vitamin A (beta-carotene), vitamin C, folic acid, iron	Stir-fry or steam; serve with a squeeze of lemon.	In the fridge with the cut ends in water. Cook within 2 days of purchase.
Broccoli	1/2 cup cooked	22	2.3	Potassium, vitamin A (beta-carotene), vitamin C; lutein, vitamin K, phosphorous	Delicious raw with a low-fat dip; also excellent steamed, stir-fried, or microwaved.	In a plastic bag in the refrigerator and use within 3 days. Broccoli rabe, actually a relative of turnips and cabbage, is good steamed or braised; it will keep for 5 days in the fridge.
Brussels sprouts	1/2 cup cooked	30	2	Potassium, vitamin A (beta-carotene), vitamin C, folic acid, phosphorous, iron, lutein	Steam or sauté for best flavor.	In the refrigerator and use within 3 days.
Cabbage	1 cup shredded	17	1.6	Vitamin C, vitamin K, lutein	For a piquant coleslaw, mix with shredded carrots, a splash of white	In the refrigerator, unwashed, and use within 3 days.

Vegetable	Amount per serving	Calories (kcal)	Fiber (g)	Rich In	Tips	Storage
					wine vinegar, and fat-free dressing. Try adding chopped red onion for extra oomph!	
Carrots	¹/₂ cup raw	26	1.8	Potassium, vitamin A (beta-carotene), lutein	Eat raw or mix into casseroles, soups, and stews.	Remove tops before refrigerating. Store, well wrapped, for up to a week.
Cauliflower	1 cup raw	25	2.5	Vitamin C	Steam, stir-fry, eat raw with a low-fat yogurt dip, or bake florets at 400° on a baking pan sprayed with cooking spray for 10 to 15 minutes.	Refrigerate, tightly wrapped, for 3 to 5 days.
Eggplant	1 cup sliced	21	2	Potassium	Broil, roast, or stir-fry. Salt eggplant before cooking to draw out any moisture.	In a cool, dry place and use within 2 days.
Green beans	1 cup	37	4	Lutein, potassium, some calcium	Stir-fry, steam or microwave	Refrigerate in plastic bag 2 to 3 days.

Vegetable	Amount per serving	Calories (kcal)	Fiber (g)	Rich In	Tips	Storage
Lettuce, romaine	1 cup shredded	8	1	Vitamin A (beta-carotene), folic acid, lutein	Great in a low-cal salad, with diced red or yellow peppers, thinly sliced fennel, minced cucumber, minced pickles, and chopped tomatoes.	Refrigerate in a plastic bag for 3 to 5 days.
Mushrooms	1 cup	17	0.8	Potassium, niacin, phosphorous	Add to stews, soups, and pastas for a "meaty" texture.	In the refrigerator in a single layer, covered with a paper towel, for up to 3 days.
Onions	1/2 cup chopped	30	1.4	Some potassium	Chill an onion before you peel it under cold water to reduce tearing. Always cook over low heat to avoid bitterness.	In a cool, dry place for up to 6 weeks.
Peppers (red, yellow, green)	1/2 cup sliced raw	20	1.3	Potassium, vitamin A (beta-carotene), vitamin C, lutein	Cut into strips and eat raw, or use in stir-fries, casseroles, and omelets.	In a plastic bag in the refrigerator for up to 1 week.
Spinach	1/2 cup cooked	20	2.2	Loaded with potassium,	Use raw in salads or	Refrigerate in a plastic bag for

Vegetable	Amount per serving	Calories (kcal)	Fiber (g)	Rich In	Tips	Storage
				vitamin A (beta-carotene), lutein; rich in calcium, iron, folic acid, vitamin E, magnesium, phosphorous	cooked in omelets and casseroles.	no more than 3 days.
Tomato	1 medium	25	1.4	Potassium, vitamin A (beta-carotene), vitamin C, lutein, lycopene, vitamin K	Stuff with tuna or egg salad prepared with fat-free mayonnaise and fresh herbs.	Store ripe tomatoes at room temperature and use within 3 days.
Zucchini (and yellow squash)	1 cup sliced raw	16	1.4	Potassium, lutein	Steam, sauté, grill, or bake this versatile vegetable, or grate and use in salads.	Refrigerate in a plastic bag for up to 5 days.

FRUITS

Fruits are typically higher in calories than vegetables because of the sugar they contain, but they are a great source of nutrients, give you energy, and keep you feeling satisfied much longer than a candy bar. Check out the table below for the details on your favorite varieties. Fresh fruits can make great snacks and are the basis for innumerable wonderful desserts.

Fruit	Amount per serving	Calories (kcal)	Fiber (g)	Rich In	Tips	Storage
Apple	1 medium	80	3.7	Some potassium	Chop and add to oatmeal and sprinkle in salads; season with cinnamon when you make fresh applesauce.	In the refrigerator or a cool, dark place, and use within 3 weeks.
Apricots	4	67	3	Potassium, vitamin A (beta-carotene)	Peel top, remove pit; chop or slice and stir into yogurts or fruit salad	In a plastic bag in the fridge 3 to 5 days.
Banana	1 medium	110	2.8	Potassium, vitamin C, magnesium, folic acid	To ripen green bananas, place in a paper bag at room temperature for a couple of days.	At room temperature until ripe, then refrigerate for up to 2 weeks (don't worry when the skin turns black).
Blueberries	1 cup	80	3.9	Vitamin C, some vitamin E	Choose firm, plump berries and avoid any that look mushy or dry.	In a moisture-proof container in the fridge for up to 5 days.
Cantaloupe	1 cup cubed	50	1	Potassium, vitamin A (beta-carotene) vitamin C, lutein	For a special dessert, fill a hollowed-out half cantaloupe with fat-free	Up to 5 days in the refrigerator.

Fruit	Amount per serving	Calories (kcal)	Fiber (g)	Rich In	Tips	Storage
					vanilla ice cream or frozen yogurt.	
Cherries	1 cup	100	3.3	Potassium, vitamin A (beta-carotene), and some vitamin C and biotin	Fresh cherries are best eaten out of hand, though you can also use them in fruit salads.	Keep covered in the refrigerator as they can absorb odors from other foods; use within 3 days.
Grapefruit, pink	1/2	40	1.6	Vitamin A (beta-carotene), vitamin C, lycopene	Try broiling a grapefruit and then sprinkling it with a little Equal.	In the refrigerator for up to 1 month.
Grapes (green and red)	3/4 cup	85	1.2	Potassium, vitamin C, lutein	Frozen grapes take longer to eat than unfrozen ones, so keep a handful in the freezer for when you want a quick, sweet snack.	In the refrigerator, unwashed; will last about 1 week.
Honeydew	1 cup	62	1	Potassium	Use in salads and fruit soups.	Up to 5 days in the refrigerator.
Kiwi	1	46	2.6	Potassium, lutein; loaded with vitamin C	Kiwi makes a terrific tenderizer for	Ripen at room temperature in a paper bag,

Fruit	Amount per serving	Calories (kcal)	Fiber (g)	Rich In	Tips	Storage
					meat, so try it in a marinade.	then store for 3 days in the fridge.
Lemon	1	22	5 (however, only juice is usually used)	Vitamin C	Jazz up salad dressings and sauces, or use to flavor a glass of sparkling water.	In the refrigerator, for up to 3 weeks.
Mango	1	130	3.6	Potassium, vitamin C, vitamin A (beta-carotene)	Pay attention to texture more than color and choose mangoes that are slightly soft.	In the refrigerator for up to 5 days.
Nectarine	1	66	2.2	Potassium, vitamin A (beta-carotene)	For a sweet dessert, broil or grill.	In the refrigerator and use within 5 days.
Orange	1	60	3.1	Potassium, vitamin C; some calcium, folic acid, lutein	Choose seedless navels rather than Valencias for snacking, as they are easier to peel.	At room temperature for 2 days or in the refrigerator for up to 2 weeks.
Peach	1	42	2	Some lutein, vitamin A (beta-carotene), potassium	Speed up ripening process by placing peaches in a	In the refrigerator for up to 5 days.

Fruit	Amount per serving	Calories (kcal)	Fiber (g)	Rich In	Tips	Storage
					paper bag with an apple or a banana.	
Pear	1	100	4	Some potassium and lutein	When making fruit salad, sprinkle pear slices with a little lemon juice to keep them from turning brown.	In the refrigerator; use within 5 days.
Pineapple	1 cup cubed	76	1.8	Vitamin C, some potassium	Pineapples don't get sweeter after harvest, so pick a ripe one with a fragrant odor and fresh-looking leaves. Avoid any with dried or yellow leaves.	Refrigerated, tightly wrapped, for 2 to 3 days.
Plum	1	40	1	Some potassium, vitamin A (beta-carotene), lutein	Soften hard plums by placing in a paper bag and leaving at room temperature for a few days.	Refrigerate in a plastic bag for 3 to 5 days.
Raspberries	1 cup	60	6	Potassium, lutein, vitamin C	Use in a fruit salad or to top yogurt.	Up to 3 days in the fridge.

Fruit	Amount per serving	Calories (kcal)	Fiber (g)	Rich In	Tips	Storage
Rhubarb	½ cup	13	2	Potassium, calcium	In sauce, combined with apples.	Up to 3 days in fridge.
Strawberries	1 cup	43	3	Potassium, vitamin C	Puree for a dessert sauce; as a frozen yogurt topping.	Up to 3 days in the fridge.
Tangerine	1	40	1.9	Vitamin C, some potassium, vitamin A (beta-carotene), lutein	Choose deeply colored tangerines that are heavy for their size and without any soft spots.	In refrigerator for up to 1 week.
Watermelon	1 cup cubed	49	0.8	Potassium, vitamin C, lutein; loaded with lycopene	Combine with cubed cantaloupe and honeydew for a colorful salad.	Up to 5 days in the refrigerator.

CEREALS, BREADS, AND CRACKERS

The next time you shop for cereal, don't get swayed by the brightly colored pictures on the front of the boxes. Instead, examine the nutrition panels and choose a cereal that has no more than 120 calories and 2 grams of fat in a ¾- to 1-cup serving. Ideally, the cereal will have 6 grams or fewer of sugar and at least 3 grams (or better yet, 5 +) of fiber per serving. Often you can get a sense of whether or not cereal contains fiber from the name on the box.

It's easy to eat more cereal than the specified serving size, so use a measuring cup until you can "eyeball" the correct amount. Since cereal gets stale quickly, be sure to store it in a container with a tightly fitting cover, or at least to fasten the top of the inner bag with a plastic "chip clip." If you have space in the fridge, cereal may also be stored there. Your other alternative is to buy the little individual packages of cereal, which also solves the serving size problem for you since you can't pour out any extra into the bowl.

Don't forget about hot cereals: traditional oatmeal makes a wonderful breakfast. If you buy the instant kinds, stick with unsweetened varieties and sweeten them yourself with fresh fruit (and perhaps cinnamon with a packet of Equal or Splenda). If you love the presweetened varieties, choose those that have 130 calories or fewer per serving. Often, the store brands are practically compatible with the national brands in terms of the number of calories per serving. Look for cereals with names like "apples and cinnamon," "blueberries and cream," and "peaches and cream." Typically, these flavored varieties have less added sugar. On the other hand, some flavored varieties add lots of sugar, thus lots of calories. For example, you'll be amazed at the calorie count of "maple and brown sugar": typically 190 per individual packet, due to the additional sugar.

Bread can be another tricky purchase. Buy varieties with at least 2 grams of fiber per slice because fiber fills you up and makes you feel fuller longer. And don't be fooled into thinking that just because a label says "wheat bread" this means you are getting whole wheat bread. "Wheat" bread is really just a blend of white and whole wheat flour. A product labeled "whole wheat" must be made from 100 percent whole wheat flour. Another good option is reduced-calorie bread, which has about 40 calories in a slice. And most brands offer more fiber than white bread for the same number of calories. This is specifically recommended for women who are following a 90/10

JOY'S PICKS

To ensure that you get a cereal low in calories and sugar with adequate fiber, shop for varieties like Complete Bran Flakes, Kellogg's All-Bran, Kashi Good Friends, Kashi GoLean, Cheerios, Barbara's Puffins, Wheaties, Total, Quaker Corn Bran, and Nabisco Shredded Wheat.

If you just *can't* give up the sugary cereals

- ◆ At least stick with cereals that have no more than 10 grams of sugar.
- ◆ Mix half a sugary cereal with half a healthier cereal. For example, equal parts of Frosted Flakes and Bran Flakes.
- ◆ Sweeten one of my healthier cereal picks with a packet of Equal or Splenda—and, of course, some fresh fruit.

When shopping for bread, keep these lower-calorie versions at 40 calories per slice in mind: Wonder Light, Arnold Bakery Light, Beefsteak Rye Light, Country Kitchen Light, Entenmann's Light, and Freihofer's Light. (Wonder Light, Arnold Bakery Light, and Country Kitchen Light also pack in 5 grams of fiber—a double bonus.)

Also look for the lower-calorie versions of hamburger rolls and hot dog buns: Wonder Light (one bun equals 80 calories), Country Kitchen Light (one bun equals 80 calories).

1,200-calorie meal plan, as well as those who are trying to keep their carbohydrate intake down. (This group includes people with diabetes, elevated triglycerides, Syndrome X, polycystic ovarian syndrome, and/or blood sugar swings.)

A typical whole wheat pita has 150 calories. If you are following a stricter calorie plan, look for the smaller ones that are 70 calories. Pirouette and Sahara are two brands that make these smaller versions. And for a few extra calories, Joseph's makes a delicious whole wheat pita for 80 calories. Stick with whole-grain varieties when you buy crackers. Choose whole wheat, multigrain, rye, oat, or cracked wheat crackers. You should also replace regular english muffins with whole wheat or oat bran. The calories remain the same, but you'll gain nutrition.

When you buy pasta, select whole-grain varieties, as these offer more fiber than white. You'll notice lots of whole wheat pastas mentioned throughout the recipe section. That's because there's no reason to cook white pasta when the whole wheat version offers a greater nutritional punch. Brown rice is more healthful than white rice and has more fiber, too. And try barley, couscous, bulgur, kasha, wheat berries, cracked wheat, quinoa, and faro. Not only will they give your dinners some variety and keep you from getting bored, but they also contain fiber and valuable phytochemicals, which are plant substances that help to promote health and wellness and potentially fight off disease.

THE DAIRY DEPARTMENT

Here's where you can stock up on all the great products that provide you with calcium, along with protein, several of the B vitamins, and vitamins A and D. Unfortunately, whole milk and whole-milk cheeses have loads of saturated fat and more overall calories than their lower-fat counterparts. In general, you want to zoom in on the low-fat or nonfat dairy products and keep a distance from the others.

The incredible array of different kinds of milk now on the market can be confusing. There's whole milk, which has a fat content of around 3.5 percent; 2 percent low-fat milk, which provides

2 percent fat and has the same nutritional value as whole milk; 1 percent milk, with 1 percent fat and even fewer calories; and nonfat (or skim) milk, which contains less than 0.2 percent fat.

I strongly recommend sticking with skim milk, SkimPlus (nonfat milk fortified with extra calcium and with a thicker consistency than skim), or 1 percent low-fat milk. If you despise the taste of skim or 1 percent in your coffee, try SkimPlus or a fat-free nondairy creamer. Low-fat soy milk is recommended for vegetarians, for those who wish to avoid all dairy products (due to casein and whey allergies, and for adults and kids with increased mucus production), and those who want to boost their intake of soy protein. Low-fat and fat-free Lactaid milk is recommended for people who are lactose-intolerant.

Cheese contributes great taste to many dishes; unfortunately, traditional varieties also contribute fat. So when choosing cheeses, stick with fat-free or low-fat, keeping in mind that there's a big difference in taste and texture depending on the variety and brand you buy. In general, fat-free sharp cheddar tastes much better than the fat-free American varieties. Among the varieties and brands I recommend prepackaged, sliced Kraft fat-free sharp cheddar, Borden fat-free sharp cheddar, and the larger loose bags of Sargento and Healthy Choice low-fat shredded cheese (all flavor varieties). And for kids and kids at heart, opt for Polly-O part-skim string cheese and Healthy Choice string cheese.

I also recommend that you pick up 1 percent low-fat cottage cheese and either low-fat or nonfat yogurt. If you're aiming to reduce your sugar intake, stick with the nonfat artificially sweetened yogurts such as Colombo Lite, Breyers Light, and Dannon Light 'n Fit. These generally have 120 calories per 8-ounce container (or 90 calories per 6-ounce container) and are significantly lower than other yogurts in carbohydrates. For a truer yogurt taste and a thicker consistency, try Total nonfat Greek yogurt at only 80 calories per 5-ounce container. And for just a few extra calories, try adding a teaspoon of your favorite preserves into any brand of plain, nonfat yogurt. Also, for folks looking for low-fat or nonfat flavored yogurt, prepared *without* any artificial sweetener, I highly recommend Stonyfield Farm.

Reduced-fat or nonfat sour cream is great for garnishing soups and spooning onto tacos and quesadillas. It's gratifying to see companies like Breakstone (which makes an excellent reduced-fat sour cream) accommodating calorie-conscious consumers by coming up with lower fat products. Try nonfat sour cream in Shepherd's Pie with Cauliflower and Turkey as well as in savory Slow-Cooker Beef Stroganoff.

EGGS AND EGG SUBSTITUTES

Eggs provide protein, vitamins, and minerals (they are an excellent source of riboflavin). In a whole egg, more than half the protein (3.5 grams) is in the white. The yolk contains the rest of the protein, all the fat (about 5 grams), and 213 milligrams of cholesterol. Thanks to the array of egg products now on the market, you can enjoy omelets, frittatas, and tarts that taste like the real thing without extra calories and dietary cholesterol. Look for AllWhites, which contains 100 percent egg whites, no fat or cholesterol, 5 grams of protein, and 25 calories per serving—equivalent to the volume of one large egg. To use in meringues and angel food cakes, you may also buy All-Whites Whippin' Whites. Egg Beaters and Smart Eggs contain 99 percent whites, along with flavors, spices, and some vitamins. A ¼-cup serving, equivalent to one egg, has 30 calories, zero fat or cholesterol, and 6 grams of protein. Since they are nearly all protein, these egg substitutes may become rubbery if overcooked, but the consistency is substantial, much like a real egg.

Of course, you don't have to buy egg substitutes to avoid the fat and cholesterol in eggs: You can simply discard the yolks and use the whites in scrambled eggs or omelets. For a thicker consistency, you can mix one whole egg with two to three egg whites. You'll never miss the extra yolks!

Eggs come in assorted sizes: jumbo, extra-large, large, medium, and small. The recipes in this book were tested with extra-large. Always buy eggs with no cracks and with clean shells. They are already washed and coated with an oil so there is no need to wash eggs. And by the way, there's absolutely no nutritional difference between white and brown eggs. Be sure to check the sell-by date and select eggs that are the closest to the shelf in the dairy case. Eggs that are near the top of a stack may not be kept as cold as they should be. Keep eggs in the refrigerator, where the temperature is below 40°, in their cartons, not on the egg racks built into some refrigerator doors. Eggs will keep (in the refrigerator in their carton) for two weeks past the sell-by date, according to the American Egg Board!

FISH AND SEAFOOD

Shop often at the fish department or your specialty fish store, for here are some of the best bargains around from the dieter's standpoint. Fish is high in flavor and naturally low in calories, and when you prepare it yourself, you can keep its natural fat content low by using plenty of spices and herbs and avoiding breading and frying. Besides being a wonderful source of protein and zinc, fish is versatile. You'll find plenty of seafood dishes to savor in the recipe section, including Citrus Fish Paillard, Moroccan Spiced Baked Fish, Italian Fish Stew, and Maple-Glazed Salmon.

Even fish that are fattier than others contain such a small amount of fat that all fish and seafood varieties are still a great nutritional choice. Plus, the type of fat found in fish is polyunsaturated and provides those heart-healthy omega-3 fatty acids that aid in digestion and help fight cardiovascular disease and maybe even cancer. Fish also contains high-quality protein, vitamins, and minerals.

The leanest fish include cod, flounder, sea bass, whiting, halibut, red snapper, haddock, mullet, perch, and shellfish such as crab, lobster, and shrimp. The fattier fish include salmon, mackerel, shad, pompano, herring, bluefish, albacore tuna, and catfish.

Frozen fish is just as nutritious and tasty as fresh and, in some instances, it may even be fresher. Be sure to avoid breaded seafood, as there is no reason to consume all those extra calories. Shrimp nearly always is shipped frozen and then defrosted before it is sold. If possible, buy it still frozen, as you can then control how and when it is thawed. Frozen shrimp also tends to be less expensive than fresh shrimp. Another money saver at the fish counter these days is salmon, so when it goes on sale, buy a fillet weighing a couple of pounds, slice it into single portions, and freeze each portion in a sealed bag.

You may also pick up some imitation crabmeat (or spend more on the real stuff) and use it to make one of the tastiest lunch recipes in the book (it's also one of the easiest): Boston Crab Salad Triangles.

When you shop for seafood, choose what looks fresh and appealing. Fish and seafood should have bright skin, bulging eyes (for whole fish), firm flesh, and no fishy smell. Steer clear of prewrapped fish, and (it goes without saying!) avoid fish counters that smell.

POULTRY

When you remove the skin, which is pure fat, poultry is one of the leanest animal protein sources around. Even if you buy poultry with the skin on, and cook it with the skin intact for added moistness, be sure to discard it before eating. The leanest poultry choices are skinless chicken breast, white meat turkey breast, Cornish game hens without the skin, duck and pheas-

Mercury Levels in Fish

Nearly all fish contains trace amounts of methylmercury, which may be dangerous and some long-lived, larger fish that feed on other fish accumulate higher levels. Shark, tilefish, swordfish, and king mackerel are the highest in mercury and should be completely avoided for now. Even tuna contains some mercury, though the mercury levels in canned and fresh tuna are about one-third of that found in shark and swordfish. I recommend limiting your consumption of tuna to two times a week. If you're unsure about the latest information on fish consumption in your area, check with your state or local health department to see if there are any special advisories on fish since official recommendations may change from time to time. You may also learn about the "Risks of Mercury in Seafood" by calling 1-888-SAFEFOOD.

ant without the skin, and extra-lean ground chicken or turkey breast. It's always a good idea to check the label to make sure it's white meat only, with no skin added. Ground poultry is a great alternative to beef for meat loaf, chili, and burgers, and you'll find plenty of recipes using both extra-lean ground turkey and chicken in these pages.

Buying ground chicken and turkey can be truly confusing, since packages in the meat case proclaim things like "97 percent fat-free" and "95 percent lean." There is no standard regulating the amount of fat that ground poultry may contain, though it is typically about 10–15 percent fat by weight. Nutrition labels aren't mandatory on ground poultry products, until a producer uses the terms "lean" or "extra-lean" to describe the products. Then a nutrition label must appear on the package and the information on the nutrition facts panel must support this claim.

Here is what you need to know before you make a ground poultry purchase. "Lean" means that a serving of approximately 3 ounces (sometimes it can range up to 4 ounces) of ground chicken or turkey has fewer than 10 grams of fat, 4.5 grams saturated fat, and 95 milligrams of cholesterol. "Extra-lean" means that a 3-ounce serving has fewer than 5 grams of fat, 2 grams of saturated fat, and 95 milligrams of cholesterol.

I strongly recommend that you never buy ground poultry below 90 percent lean (or 90 percent fat-free). Ideally, you should always opt for the 95–99 percent fat-free. (Remember, it may also say 95–99 percent "extra-lean.") If your grocer does not carry "extra-lean," then my second choice is to purchase 90–95 percent lean or fat-free.

When cooked, the extra-lean meat might seem a little drier, but once you add some seasonings and sauce, it tastes just fine. For example, in Extra-Lean Turkey Chili, you mix extra-lean ground turkey with delicious, flavorful ingredients for a wonderful, filling main course.

STORING GROUND POULTRY

Once you get that ground chicken or turkey home, pop it right into the fridge.

Uncooked ground chicken or turkey may be stored for one to two days in the fridge or three to four months in the freezer.

Cooked ground chicken or poultry will keep for three to four days or two to three months in the freezer.

For additional information on food safety, call the USDA Meat and Poultry Hot Line at 1-800-535-4555.

Along the same guidelines, when buying boneless chicken or turkey cutlets and breasts, stick with the extra-lean, meaning 95–100 percent lean or fat-free. If possible, choose a product that is closer to 100 percent fat-free and look for unbreaded, of course. With so many great marinated poultry products on the market today, you'll have no problem choosing a healthful variety. Perdue makes excellent marinated boneless chicken breast products that you just put in the oven. You'll also find store brand versions at your local grocery store and at popular price clubs.

LOW-CALORIE EASY MARINADE

To make an easy marinade for boneless chicken breasts, whisk together 2 tablespoons olive oil, 2 tablespoons lemon juice, 2 teaspoons Dijon mustard, 1 minced scallion, 1 minced clove garlic, ¼ teaspoon salt, and a dash of pepper. Pour over the chicken and marinate for at least 1 hour before grilling.

Chicken nuggets are very high in fat and calories. Instead of buying nuggets in the supermarket, try the recipes for Rainbow Chicken Nuggets and Crunchy Chicken Strips with Honey Mustard Sauce. You'll also find a wide variety of soy nugget alternatives in the vegetarian section of many grocery stores.

One of the trickier purchases in the supermarket is luncheon meats. However, they are a better choice than the typical restaurant sandwich, which contains anywhere from 4 to 66 grams of fat and from 350 to 1,000 calories. Clearly, you can save plenty of calories (not to mention money!) when you buy the proper cold cuts and make your own lunch. If you want a low-fat sandwich, turkey or chicken breast is a good bet, since 4 ounces of meat have just 7 grams of fat. If the meat is processed, cut back to 2 ounces to keep your sodium intake low.

When shopping for poultry cold cuts, keep in mind that brand-name companies go out of their way to advertise when a product is "extra-lean," fat-free, or low-fat. Once again, look for packages that read 95–100 percent fat-free or lean (this will ensure that the cold cuts have no more than 4 grams of fat per serving). Also remember that the sodium levels are often very high in processed cold cuts. This may be the time you want to skip the high-sodium pickle on the side and have some crunchy baby carrots instead. If sodium is an issue, shop for brands that have 500 milligrams of sodium or fewer per 2-ounce serving. And of

JOY'S PICKS

The following "extra-lean" varieties of poultry brands meet my criteria, but remember that the latter three brands also make the full-fat versions so read the packages carefully: Healthy Choice, Butterball, Louis Rich, and Oscar Mayer.

course, whenever you have the opportunity, buy freshly sliced turkey breast at the deli counter, which is equally lean and generally lower in sodium than the processed varieties. Also, for a little extra effort, you can enjoy your own freshly prepared chicken or turkey. On a night you're cooking dinner, go ahead and bake an extra breast in the oven, then slice thinly for sandwiches and salads the following day.

MEATS: BEEF, VEAL, LAMB, PORK

Overall, there's good news about beef: In some instances, it's bred to be much leaner than it was years ago, with less outer fat and less marbling. If you like beef but want to avoid all the saturated fat, you can have your beef and eat it too, so long as you shop carefully and choose the leaner cuts. Select beef that is bright red with very light visible marbling. Press the meat in its package with your fingers to make sure that it is firm.

The USDA grades all beef according to tenderness, juiciness, and flavor, and these qualities all relate to the amount of marbling (which basically is fat) in the animal. The highest grade is "prime," followed by "choice" and "select." Both "choice" and "select" have less marbling and may be tougher than prime meat, but they can be made more tender with the proper cooking techniques. Cuts from the chuck and the round, which are active muscles, are also leaner and tougher than the loin. But marinating these cuts makes them much more tender.

Well-marbled meat is the juiciest and tenderest, but also the highest in fat. That's the meat you should avoid buying. A 4-ounce well-marbled portion of broiled T-bone steak, for instance, can have 24 grams of fat and much of it the artery-clogging type. Not only is that too much fat, but this cut of meat also is too high in calories.

Although lean cuts of beef aren't as easy to find as lean cuts of poultry, they are definitely available. Buy beef that is at least 90 percent fat-free or 90 percent lean and contains 10 grams or fewer of fat per serving. Or look for even leaner cuts, such as 95 percent lean or more. Again, since leaner cuts can be tougher than well-marbled meats, check below for tips on tenderizing them. Also, check out the delicious Herb-Marinated Flank Steak in the recipe section.

HOW TO TENDERIZE LEANER CUTS OF MEAT

Marinate flank steak in low-sodium soy sauce, rice vinegar, and garlic, then grill or broil it and slice it across the grain, for an entrée that will satisfy the most diehard meat lover.

To give flank steak a southwestern flavor, mix 2 tablespoons olive oil, 2 tablespoons red wine vinegar, 1 teaspoon sugar, 2 teaspoons dried oregano, 1 teaspoon chili powder, ½ teaspoon garlic powder, ½ teaspoon salt, and a dash of freshly ground pepper. Prick the meat with a fork in several places, then pour the marinade over and allow to sit for 8 hours in the fridge, turn the meat occasionally, then grill or broil.

Ordinary ground meat tends to have a fat content greater than 20 percent—that's too much fat and too many calories. I suggest using extra-lean ground turkey in most of your recipes. But certainly if you are a beef lover, look for extra-lean ground sirloin, which has a rich flavor. If you have to buy ground beef with the higher fat content, be sure to rinse or blot after cooking to get rid of any extra fat. Always fully drain the fat from cooked meat prior to adding it to a marinara sauce or using in tacos or chili. To take it one step further, you may want to consider placing the meat into a strainer and rinsing with hot tap water. In this case, add seasonings after rinsing.

Veal is defined as the meat of a calf up to the age of three months or maybe slightly older. (Once it's six months old, veal is called "baby beef.") Unlike beef, veal is low in fat and has little or no marbling. All the veal cuts except those from the loin, rib, and leg are good for stewing and braising since they're so low in fat. While cuts of veal are typically lean, keep in mind that veal chops can be very fatty around the bone. That's why this is everyone's favorite part of the chop! A great option is the veal tip, which is sliced and pounded to become veal scallops.

Like beef and veal, the USDA grades lamb, and the tenderest lamb tends to have the most marbling. Lamb has five USDA grades, all based on the proportion of fat to lean meat. Most of the lamb sold to consumers is choice. When shopping for lamb, check the color. Generally, the darker the color, the older the animal—not as desirable and likelier to be less tender.

Weight is another factor to keep in mind. A 10-pound leg of lamb will be stronger flavored and slightly tougher than a smaller leg. For a dinner party, you may want to go for a different part of the lamb. Remember that some parts of the lamb can be fatty: the breast is fatty though flavorful, for example, while the saddle contains the tender and very well-marbled sirloin. With a moderate fat content, lamb shoulder is juicier than leaner cuts such as lamb flank. Unfortunately, it tends to be a little tougher as there's less fat, and it's typically sold ground. One good lean cut of lamb is the foreshank, which may be braised to delicious, melting-off-the-bone tenderness. Also try grilled kebabs, in which chunks of boneless lamb sirloin alternate with vegetables on a skewer, and the Indian Lamb Stew.

You might think of pork as high-fat meat, but it's much leaner today than it used to be. Compared to a decade ago, pork is higher in protein and lower in calories. Still, not all cuts are lean.

Bacon, for instance, has about 3.5 grams of fat per slice. You're better off substituting an ounce of lean cured ham, which has fewer than 2 grams of fat.

Processed meat products such as sausage, bologna, salami, and hot dogs get between 70 and 80 percent of their total calories from fat, so steer clear of them as much as possible.

Bacon, Hot Dogs, and Sausage: Sometimes You Just Have to Eat Them! When you want to indulge, check out the tables that follow. These provide rules of thumb and brand-name suggestions to guide you toward the best bets in bacon, hot dogs, and sausages.

While regular bacon is too high in fat (typically 14 grams per ounce), the following brands offer much leaner alternatives.

If you love hot dogs, keep in mind that an ordinary 2-ounce dog can contain as much as 15 grams of fat, almost half of that saturated. I recommend the following brands, all of which are so low in fat and calories that you could have two at either lunch or dinner. Of course, you'll have to

Lean Bacon Alternatives

Brand	Amount	Calories (kcal)	Fat (g)	Protein (g)	Fiber (g)	Sodium (mg)
Applegate Farms turkey bacon	1 slice	38	<1	3	0	306
Butterball turkey bacon	1 slice	23	1.7	1.3	0	120
Canadian pork bacon most varieties	1 slice	43	2	6	0	358
Hormel Canadian-style bacon	1 slice	34	1.5	4.5	0	284
Jennie-O extra-lean turkey bacon	1 slice	20	0.5	3	0	130
Louis Rich turkey bacon	1 slice	35	2.5	2	0	180
Shelton's turkey bacon	1 slice	25	1	3	0	210
Yorkshire (Wellshire) Farms turkey bacon	1 slice	20	0.5	3	0	180

Lean Hot Dog Alternatives

Brand	Amount	Calories (kcal)	Fat (g)	Protein (g)	Fiber (g)	Sodium (mg)
Ball Park fat-free franks	1 frank	50	0	6	0	490
Butterball fat-free franks	1 frank	40	0	5	0	490
Eckrich lite franks	1 frank	100	6	5	0	420
Empire Kosher turkey franks	1 frank	100	8	6	0	540
Hebrew National 97% fat-free franks	1 frank	45	1.5	6	0	400
Oscar Mayer fat-free hot dogs	1 frank	40	0	6	0	490
Select Healthy Choice franks	1 frank	70	2.5	6	0	440

limit bread consumption, so that you don't consume more carbs than are recommended on your personal 90/10 plan.

Look for sausages that are labeled "97 percent fat-free," "97 percent lean," "low-fat" or "fat-free." If the label on a sausage just says "reduced fat," it may contain 25 percent less fat than a version that's very high in fat, which isn't good enough.

VEGETARIAN PROTEIN OPTIONS

If you don't eat meat, you can flavor omelets, chilies, and casseroles with soy products and impart a satisfying taste and texture. Even if you are a meat eater, you can still enjoy some of these delicious meatless options. Another reason to get acquainted with soy-based vegetarian fare is that soy has been shown to be beneficial to your overall health.

You may substitute soy nuggets for chicken nuggets in family meals—most kids can't tell the difference. And most of the vegan (nondairy) vegetarian foods are automatically low in saturated fat. Just try to pick packages that have fewer than 400 milligrams of sodium per serving. Choose among the wide array of vegetarian link sausages, soy crumbles, tofu hot dogs, and veggie burgers.

Leaner Sausages Alternatives

Brand	Amount	Calories (kcal)	Fat (g)	Protein (g)	Fiber (g)	Sodium (mg)
Amy's chicken sausage	1 link (2 oz)	100	4.5	13	0	410
Bilinski's chicken sausage	1 link (2 oz)	70–90	3–5	9	0–1	270–300
Butterball fat-free smoked sausage	1 link (2 oz)	60	0	9	0	680
Casual Gourmet chicken sausage	1 link (3 oz)	110	2.5	19	0	640
Healthy Choice breakfast links	3 small links (2 oz)	70	3	8	0	480
smoked links	1 link (2 oz)	80	2.5	7	0	480
Jimmy Dean 97% fat-free breakfast sausage	1 slice (⅙ of roll) (2.5 oz)	90	2	11	0	410
Shadybrook Farms						
breakfast turkey sausage	2 links (2.5 oz)	80	4	10	0	480
turkey sausage	1 link (3 oz)	90	4	12	0	450
Yorkshire Farms (Wellshire Farms)						
roasted turkey	1 link (2 oz)	70	3.5	8	0	460
smoked pork	1 link (2 oz)	130	6	17	0	350
smoked turkey	1 link (2 oz)	60	3	9	0	280

There are many different varieties of soy burgers, and the nutrition information varies depending on which one you choose. In general, these burgers can provide a decent amount of soy protein for a small amount of calories. You'll also find delicious soy-based "chick" patties, vegetarian sausages, and nuggets.

Vegetarian Burgers

Brand	Amount	Calories (kcal)	Fat (g)	Protein (g)	Fiber (g)	Sodium (mg)
Amy's Burgers	1 patty					
California		130	5	6	5	430
Texas		120	2.5	12	3	350
Chicago		160	5	10	3	390
American		120	3	10	3	390
Boca Burgers	1 patty					
original		90	1	13	4	350
grilled veggie		80	1	13	5	300
cheese		130	6	13	4	420
flame grilled		110	4	14	4	370
Gardenburgers	1 patty					
original		110	3	6	3	560
flame grilled		120	4	14	4	300
Veggie Medley		90	0	5	3	280
Morningstar Farms burgers	1 patty	80–150	0–6	10–18	2–5	300–400

Vegetarian Sausages

Brand	Amount	Calories (kcal)	Fat (g)	Protein (g)	Fiber (g)	Sodium (mg)
Boca Sausage Links	1 sausage (large)					
Italian		130	6	11	3	990
smoked		130	5	12	2	890
bratwurst		130	7	11	2	870
Morningstar Farms breakfast links	2 links (small)	60	2	8	2	340

Vegetarian Soy-Based "Chick" Patties

Brand	Amount	Calories (kcal)	Fat (g)	Protein (g)	Fiber (g)	Sodium (mg)
Mon Cuisine chick patty	1 patty	100	2.5	7	3	290
Morningstar Farms chik patties	1 patty	150	6	9	2	570
Worthington crispy chick patties	1 patty	150	6	9	2	440
fillets	2 pieces	180	9	16	4	650

Vegetarian Nuggets

Brand	Amount	Calories (kcal)	Fat (g)	Protein (g)	Fiber (g)	Sodium (mg)
Boca chick'n nuggets	4 nuggets	190	7	16	2	570
Mon Cuisine chicken nuggets	4 nuggets	140	4	12	4	380
Morningstar Farms chik nuggets	4 nuggets	180	6	13	5	590
Veggie Patch chick'n nuggets	5 nuggets	160	4	15	2	600

FROZEN ENTRÉES AND SOUPS

For days when you just don't have time to cook, it's tempting to fall into the trap of ordering in pizza or Chinese food. But the supermarket has some wonderful and healthy foods that are low in fat and calories, and ready in a matter of minutes. Let's review frozen entrées and canned soups, which should be stocked in everyone's freezer and pantry for those last-minute meal options.

Choose canned soup that is low in fat and calories and has just a moderate amount of sodium. Let's face it: Even though a serving size generally says 1 cup of soup, most people eat the whole can's worth. So seek out soups that, per can, don't contain more than 300 calories, 800 milligrams of sodium, and 6 grams of fat. Brands I like are Healthy Choice, Health Valley, Campbell's Healthy

Request, and Progresso 99% Fat Free. Most varieties of these brands make the grade.

The simplest rule of thumb for buying frozen foods is to choose according to which 90/10 plan you are on. If you're following the 1,200-calorie plan, you get 350 calories for dinner, so select a frozen entrée with 300 calories and 10 grams or fewer of fat. That way, you can supplement with a salad or a cup of steamed vegetables. Ideally, the frozen entrée should contain no more than 800 milligrams of sodium. If you're on the 1,400-calorie plan, look for entrées that are 400 calories or fewer, and if you're on the 1,600- to 2,000-calorie plan, buy entrées that are 500 calories or fewer. A few brands that I recommend are Healthy Choice, Lean Cuisine, Amy's, and Smart Ones.

DRESSINGS, MARINADES, AND CONDIMENTS

Salad Dressings Pour regular bottled salad dressing over your low-cal greens and your salad's calorie count skyrockets into the hundreds. That's because 1 tablespoon of dressing typically has 100 calories, and it's easy to use 4 or more tablespoons on a regular salad. Although many dressings are made with olive oil, which is the unsaturated healthy fat, for weight management we still need to worry about our total calories, no matter where they come from. That's the bad news.

The good news is that there are many wonderful light and fat-free salad dressings on the market. The low-fat dressings cut the calorie count of your salad in half, while the fat-free dressings can contain as few as 5 per tablespoon (sometimes zero, though taste can be compromised). There is a wide array of good brands on the market; your rule of thumb for store-bought dressing is that it should contain 30 calories or fewer for 2 tablespoons (serving size for salad dressing is generally listed as 2 tablespoons on the label).

If you have time, another great idea is to make your own dressing. It can taste better than anything you pour out of a bottle and allows you to control the proportion of oil to vinegar. The classic vinaigrette dressing is a mixture of these two: the oil can be a neutral vegetable oil like canola or extra-virgin olive oil, or a specialty oil like walnut, peanut, flaxseed, or sesame.

Oils Supermarkets stock so many different kinds of oil today you probably won't even need to visit a specialty store. Canola oil is a good all-around choice for dressings because it has a light flavor. It's monounsaturated and good for stir-fries since it doesn't dominate the food. Extra-virgin olive oil is a monounsaturated oil with a fruity flavor; it is good for salad dressings. Don't be fooled by the terms "light" and "extra-light." Light olive oil contains the same amount of beneficial monounsaturated fat as regular olive oil—and the same number of calories. "Light" and "extra-light" simply refer to the taste. Use less-pricey regular olive oil for everything besides stir-fries and salad dressings.

Peanut oil, also monounsaturated, is especially good for stir-fries because it has a high smoke point, the stage at which heated oil starts to give off smoke and disagreeable odors, and produces an unpleasant flavor in the food. Flaxseed oil gives you plenty of healthful omega-3s, but it also has a somewhat heavier taste. Safflower oil is a light, all-purpose oil without much taste; like peanut oil, it has a high smoke point. Sesame oil, which is polyunsaturated, is rich and light, so you can get a lot of flavor with just a drizzle. Since it is expensive, most people do not use it as a cooking oil. Nut oils, such as walnut, are recommended for salad dressings because their strong flavor means you'll use less.

Vinegars While a classic vinaigrette salad dressing is two parts oil to one part vinegar, this formula's not set in stone. Buy the best-quality balsamic vinegar you can find, and you will require far less oil.

LOW-CALORIE VINAIGRETTE

Whisk together ½ clove crushed garlic, a pinch of salt, 1 tablespoon water, 2 teaspoons balsamic vinegar, and 2 tablespoons red wine vinegar. Gradually add 2 tablespoons extra-virgin olive oil, and whisk mixture until creamy. This makes about ¼ cup of dressing, enough for 4 people.

Add ½ teaspoon honey and ¼ teaspoon dried mustard and you've got a great honey-mustard vinaigrette.

Stock your kitchen with a few different kinds of vinegar so you can vary the flavor of salad dressings and not get bored. Some to try are rice vinegar, sherry vinegar (especially Spanish sherry vinegar, which has a woody flavor and is an excellent stand-in for balsamic vinegar), and white wine vinegar. You could also use red wine vinegar, though white wine vinegar makes prettier vinaigrette.

Boost the flavor of a homemade salad dressing by adding some chopped garlic, minced shallots or other fresh herbs, or Dijon mustard. These contribute flavor without adding much in the way of calories. All homemade dressings are best served immediately, but they'll keep for a couple of days, tightly covered, in the refrigerator.

Marinades and Miscellaneous Both catsup and mustard, as well as bottled marinades, should contain no more than 30 calories in 1 tablespoon (or 10 calories in 1 teaspoon). Be suspicious of fancy, delicious looking marinades, which can contain a lot of fat and sodium. When you buy teriyaki sauce, always make sure it's the "light" variety, which indicates that it is low in sodium. Ditto with soy sauce. Good choices for mustard are Grey Poupon and Gulden's, which contain 30 calories in 2 tablespoons. Heinz catsup, with 15 calories in a tablespoon, works well in marinades and dressings. For mayonnaise, stick with a brand that has no more than 30 calories per tablespoon. I like Hellmann's (in parts of the U.S. also known as "Best") Just 2 Good, with 25 calories in 1 tablespoon. And for jams, jellies, and preserves, opt for 30 calories or fewer per tablespoon. I recommend Smucker's Low Sugar (25 calories, 5 grams sugar per tablespoon) and Smucker's Light Sugar Free preserves (10 calories, 0 grams sugar per tablespoon).

Also, if you really love a particular marinade or condiment, don't automatically think you have to part with it. If its calorie content is too high, think of this as a red flag to be on guard about using too much.

SEASONINGS AND FRESH HERBS

Definitely include herbs on your shopping list. Whether fresh or dried, herbs allow you to infuse flavor into just about any dish without adding any calories. When you use dried herbs, crush them in your hand before adding to a food, as this helps to release their flavor. A good rule of thumb is that 1 teaspoon of dried herbs is equivalent to 1 tablespoon of fresh herbs. Be sure to add fresh herbs at the end of the cooking time, as their delicate flavor can be destroyed by heat. You may add dried herbs as a dish cooks because they need a longer exposure to heat in order to get the maximum flavor. Store fresh herbs in the fridge in a plastic bag for no more than a week, or freeze them for up to 3 months and use them in cooked dishes. Keep dried herbs in a cool, dark cupboard in tightly covered containers. Remember: They don't last forever. Discard dried herbs after a year.

Cooking with Herbs

Herbs can turn an ordinary dish into something extra special.

Basil: With its slightly minty flavor, it's excellent in salads, Italian meals, pasta dishes, and eggs.

Bay leaf: Use in dried form to flavor soups, stews, and sauces. Be sure to remove before serving, as bay leaves can be a choking hazard.

Chervil: This mild but distinctively flavored herb is good with fish, eggs, salads, and soups. With a flavor like tarragon, chervil may be substituted for tarragon. In a pinch, use parsley if you can't find chervil.

Chives: These have an onionlike flavor that makes them a nice addition to soups, eggs, and salads. Avoid dried chives: Unlike some herbs, the dried variety of chives just isn't satisfactory.

Cilantro: Sometimes called Chinese parsley or fresh coriander, it's becoming increasingly popular thanks to its slightly peppery, very aromatic flavor. Used sparingly, it lends a unique flavor to many Asian, Mexican, and Caribbean dishes.

Dill: Both fresh and dried dill weed impart an almost lemony taste to fish, salads, sauces, and vegetables.

Mint: It's used in both savory and sweet dishes, and both the dried and fresh varieties are very flavorful. Spearmint is slightly more delicate in flavor than peppermint.

Oregano: A relative of marjoram and thyme, this aromatic herb is almost a necessity in Italian cooking. Try it with any dish that calls for tomatoes, and use on roasted chicken.

Parsley: As a garnish and a flavor, this herb is extremely versatile and is delicious with seafood, poultry, pasta, and omelets. Curly leaf parsley isn't quite as flavorful as Italian parsley, which is also called flat-leaf parsley.

Rosemary: Very aromatic and strongly flavored, it brings out the flavor in roasted meat, poultry, potatoes, fish, and stews. The dried version holds its flavor well.

Sage: Chicken goes very well with sage, which has a taste somewhat reminiscent of mint. Be sure to use sparingly, as this has a strong flavor. It's wonderful in salad dressings and on some vegetables. Try fresh sage with carrots, zucchini, or butternut squash.

Tarragon: With a flavor that is reminiscent of licorice, this herb's essential in French cooking. Use with a gentle hand as it has a strong flavor. When you can't find fresh, dried is a good substitute.

Thyme: Minty, lemony, and light, it's excellent with chicken, on roasted vegetables, in soups, and with seafood.

Fun Foods

When it comes to the little fun indulgences that offer us comfort, satisfy our cravings, and give us a little psychological boost, we all have our own must-haves that range from double chocolate ice cream to salted cashews (my favorite!), from freshly baked cookies to chips and dip. My rule of thumb for a fun food is always 250 calories or fewer and it doesn't have to be sweet. The recipe section contains Oven-Baked French Fries, Guacamole, and a dynamite Hot Artichoke Dip.

The fact of the matter, though, is that often our favorite "treat" foods are the very same foods that act as triggers, causing us to overindulge even when we're perfectly aware of what we're doing. The last thing you want is for the foods that you initially eat to feel good to turn into foods that make you feel guilty.

I certainly don't have to tell you which treats you should eat as part of your meal plan. That's up to you. However, I spend the majority of my time coaching people on the 90 percent healthy and 10 percent fun foods philosophy, and I do need to warn you about the importance of identifying your own trigger foods and then keeping them out of your house. If you can't have a box of cookies around without sneaking it into the bedroom on occasion and polishing off a dozen (or more) just to make yourself feel better about something, buy single-serving cookies or skip the cookies entirely and instead buy individual bags of microwave light popcorn. If a canister of whipped cream beckons you every time you open the refrigerator to the point where you're squirting it on everything and even eating it by the spoonful, admit to yourself that you didn't really buy it for your child's hot chocolate—and stop keeping it around. Let's face it, your kids aren't the ones who are really going to miss it! And if you've got kids in the house who are clamoring for everything from cupcakes to ice cream to soda, do yourself a favor and buy them the foods you hate. I once urged one of my chocoholic clients to give out Sour Warheads and Smartees on Halloween because she wouldn't touch the leftovers.

If an entire pint of ice cream becomes one serving, avoid it entirely and instead stick with single-serving ice cream pops. (Häagen-Dazs sorbet, Smart Ones fudge pops, Yoplait fudge pops, Edy's [also known as "Dryers" in parts of the U.S.] pops, Sharon's Sorbet pops, or Silhouette fudge bars and flying saucers are all delicious and automatically portion-controlled.) Another strategy is to pick up a small soft-serve (to go) of low-fat frozen yogurt from your local shop.

Furthermore, if you're a polish-off-an-open-bag kind of person, you clearly shouldn't be buying any of your favorite foods that have multiple servings in one large bag. And you probably should keep no more than one day's fun food allotment within easy reach.

One of my clients can't stop eating chips once the bag is opened. However, she can't seem to live without them. Thus, I make sure that she buys only small single-serving bags—and that she keeps them well out of sight!

If you have no trouble resisting your favorite foods when they are sitting in your cupboards (in other words, you're fine with knowing how much you're allotted each day, sticking to that portion, and letting the rest of the box sit in your kitchen), you're far ahead of the game. Some people can do this with anything and everything, managing just fine with all kinds of tempting foods.

Here's something else to think about. Some people don't have to shop for these fun foods— they automatically come up. If you have a hectic lifestyle where you're constantly on the go, "extra items" may surface at restaurants, business meetings, dinners out, and even your kids' play dates. In other words, they are built into your schedule. If this describes your routine, you can enjoy one or two cocktails at a business dinner, split a dessert with a friend in a restaurant, or legally nibble on Goldfish while at your toddler's play date. But *don't* go looking for extra snacks to load into your shopping cart!

Whatever strategies you employ, once you've reached an understanding with yourself about which foods you can and just can't have in the house, it's that much easier to stick with your meal plan and keep up your resolve. Recognizing the weak chinks in your armor will gird you for an important battle: not nibbling on your favorite foods just because they're there.

As you now know, this chapter provides many best bets in brand-name foods. On your shopping excursions, you'll certainly find that there are hundreds and hundreds of food items that weren't mentioned that can fit beautifully into your weight-management program. It's important

Nutrition Label Cheat Sheet

Calorie free: Fewer than 5 calories per serving.
Low-calorie: 40 calories or fewer for most food items; 120 calories or fewer for main dish products.
Reduced-calorie: Must contain at least 25 percent fewer calories than the regular version of that food item.

Fat-free: Fewer than 0.5 gram of fat per serving.
Low-fat: 3 grams of fat (or fewer) per serving.
Reduced-fat: At least 25 percent less fat per serving than the original version of a food product.
Saturated fat-free: Fewer than 0.5 gram of saturated fat per serving.
Low in saturated fat: 1 gram or fewer per serving, or no more than 10 percent of calories coming from saturated fat.
Reduced saturated fat: At least 25 percent less saturated fat than the original version.

Cholesterol-free: Fewer than 2 milligrams of cholesterol and 2 grams (or fewer) of saturated fat per serving.
Low-cholesterol: 20 milligrams (or fewer) of cholesterol and 2 grams (or fewer) of saturated fat per serving.

Sodium-free: Fewer than 5 milligrams of sodium per serving.
Low-sodium: 140 milligrams (or fewer) of sodium per serving.
Reduced sodium: At least 25 percent less sodium than the original food version.

Organic: Must be 100 percent organic or at least 95 percent organic by weight.
Made with organic: Must be at least 70 percent organic.
The word "organic" on the ingredients panel: When less than 70 percent of the overall content is organic, the company is permitted to detail only individual organic items.

Daily percent value: How much of a day's recommended amount for certain nutrient is supplied in one serving of the food. Daily percent value is based on a 2,000-calorie diet.

for you as a diet-conscious consumer to learn and understand how to compare food items by their nutritional label. Above is a "cheat sheet" to help you continue to shop smart and to stake out the best buys.

Now that you've learned to be a shrewd, savvy shopper, it's time for a quick course in how to cook healthfully. In the next chapter, I'll teach you the right way to steam and braise, how to eyeball the correct serving size, and how to substitute one ingredient for another.

Three

Cooking ABC's

You've arrived home from the supermarket, unpacked the contents of every bag into the cupboards and the refrigerator, and looked at the labels on the various foods you've selected. You're ready to get started! But before you open that fridge or turn that oven dial, arm yourself with as much knowledge as possible about low-fat, low-calorie cooking.

This chapter helps you become perfectly comfortable in your kitchen, provides guidelines for portion control, and teaches the different cooking techniques you need to know for weight management. You'll learn all the basics: how to steam, stir-fry, poach, braise, roast, and more.

Of course, all the recipes in this book guide you through all the steps of meal preparation and ensure that each dish you cook is delicious. But there are days you want to create something special on your own, and this chapter provides you with all the necessary know-how so you'll feel confident and relaxed in the kitchen.

Knowing how to make a simple, nutritious vegetable dish or a satisfying roast turkey enables you to turn out balanced, filling, and beautiful meals and snacks for yourself and your family every time. Getting to know your ingredients—from meat, poultry, and vegetables to oils and spices—makes you a better cook and, in the long run, saves you time and effort in the kitchen. And learning how to play up foods that are naturally low in fat and calories means that you're able to prepare meals that your whole family will love and that will enable you to manage your weight.

What's more portion distortion has become so prevalent that many of us think nothing of eating a giant 800-calorie bagel for breakfast or a 12-ounce T-bone steak for dinner. To help you get back on track, I teach you how to eyeball portions so that you are eating reasonable serving sizes, a crucial strategy in your weight-loss success.

Portion Distortion

Megaportions—and who doesn't love 'em?—are one of the chief reasons we have so much trouble losing weight. It's bad enough that we overindulge when we eat out, but then we come home and, without an understanding of portion control, mimic what we see in restaurants.

Steakhouses routinely boast that their T-bones weigh close to a pound, and fast-food restaurants supersize drinks and french fries to the point where an order can easily exceed 1,000 calories. A slice of carrot cake at one popular restaurant chain weighs nearly a pound and is large enough to serve as dessert for an entire family (it contains 1,800 calories!). And coffee shops stock muffins that weigh in at 800 or 900 calories.

We also tend to use our plates to determine appropriate portion size. I once asked a client how she gauged portion size at home. She replied simply, "When each plate is filled up."

How can we start once again to recognize what really is a reasonable serving size? Get to know what it looks like: A cup of dry cereal is about the size of a baseball. And for other starches such as pasta, rice, couscous, and mashed potatoes, here is a great rule of thumb: A ½-cup serving (which is the way to go for most sedentary women looking to lose weight) is 3 heaping tablespoons. For people with a little more leeway with starch calories, a 1-cup serving is 6 heaping tablespoons.

A 1½-ounce serving of cheddar cheese is about the size of a C battery, and a 3-ounce serving of meat is about the size of a deck of cards (both length and height) or the palm of your hand. Five ounces sizes up to about 1½ decks of cards, or your palm up to the first knuckle.

Of course, most of us don't take along a deck of cards when we eat out, but you get the idea. When you eat out, just guestimate the correct portion size. Then portion out that much of your serving, push the rest to the side of the plate, and ask for a doggy bag to take it home. Once you get good at eyeballing at home by measuring, you'll know what restaurant portions constitute a reasonable size.

From a psychological standpoint, a lot of people need to know that they can eat unlimited amounts of some foods. Although 1 cup of vegetables is included in my meal plans, this is where you have carte blanche to inflate the portion size. That's because megaportions of non-starchy vegetables will not impede your weight loss. So go ahead, except, as previously stated, with the more calorically dense veggies: peas, corn, lima beans, potatoes, and winter squash.

You can also learn to painlessly downsize your helpings by eating from your plate, rather than from a package, so that you know precisely how much you are getting. Keep in mind that less looks like more when you use smaller dishes, plates, and cups. And meat doesn't have to take up the largest space on the plate. For effective, long-lasting weight management, let vegetables play a starring role in your meal. Now you will learn many different ways to prepare them, and by the end of this chapter you will know that vegetables do not have to be boring and bland.

Becoming Savvy in the Kitchen

Even if you're not a seasoned chef, you can become a low-calorie cooking expert. This chapter provides the best cooking advice for how to master flavorful methods of food preparation that don't add calories. It's your definitive guide to cooking light, a reference that you'll find yourself turning to time and again.

Let's start with vegetables. When you're in need of a quick energy boost, want to snack on something crunchy and crisp, or need a low-calorie, high-volume filler, vegetables are a wise choice. You can use veggies in so many ways: grate them and add them to meat loaf, lasagna, omelets, and mashed potatoes. Add to a thin-crust pizza for a "deluxe" pie, or load them onto your dinner plate so that your 3-ounce portion of meat doesn't look in the least bit skimpy. Vegetables are not only a boon to anyone who's trying to lose weight, they're also loaded with all the good things our bodies need—fiber, vitamins, phytochemicals, and antioxidants. Vegetables are naturally low in fat, which makes them a double-bonus food.

So how can you boost the flavor, keep them from getting boring, and keep down the fat content? With the proper cooking methods. Obvious ones to avoid are deep frying and sautéing with lots of oil or butter. How you want your vegetable to turn out will help you determine how to cook it. When you cook vegetables in a minimum amount of oil over high heat, they emerge crisp and tempting. Alternatively, if you cook them over low heat with liquid, they become tender and soft.

Steaming

Besides being quick, this method allows you to serve veggies that are flavorful but not water-logged. You need an inexpensive metal steamer to hold the vegetables out of the water in the cooking pot. You simply bring the water to the boil, add the vegetables in their steamer basket, cover, and cook over medium heat until they are tender (but not mushy). Be sure the water doesn't touch the food and, of course, keep your eye on the pot so it doesn't boil dry. The best veggies for steaming are green beans, zucchini, summer squash, broccoli, and cauliflower.

You can bump up the flavor in cooked vegetables by adding some minced onion, shallots, or garlic to the cooking liquid. Herbs like parsley also lend flavor. Sprinkle some on top after cooking. If you like a spicier dish, a sprinkle of red pepper flakes can increase the heat of a vegetable. Another seasoning option is to top cooked vegetables with one to two teaspoons of freshly grated Parmesan cheese.

STEAMED CAULIFLOWER

Cut up a head of cauliflower into florets. Place the florets in a metal steamer in a pot of simmering water, making sure the water doesn't touch the vegetables. Steam 8 to 12 minutes or until done, then remove the vegetables immediately to a serving bowl. Season with 1 teaspoon melted, reduced-fat, soft tub margarine; ½ teaspoon garlic powder; ½ teaspoon sea salt; and freshly ground black pepper. Sprinkle with 1 tablespoon chopped fresh parsley. Serves 4.

Microwaving

Similar to steaming, microwaving allows you to retain nutrients, flavors, and colors; another advantage is a short cooking time. Microwave cooking also lets you skip butter or oil and maximize flavor through seasonings. Because of their high water content, a number of vegetables cook up especially nicely in a microwave. Just about anything goes, from artichokes to sugar snap peas, and you can quickly wilt fresh spinach to serve as a hot side dish.

Winter squash and potatoes cook much more quickly with this method than in a conventional oven; always be sure to pierce the skin or outer membrane before placing them into the microwave so they don't explode. The best way to microwave fresh veggies is to place a small amount of water in the dish with the food, cover with a microwave-safe dish (venting to create a hole for steam to escape), and cook at 100 percent power. Read the labels to find out the cooking instructions for frozen vegetables. About halfway through the cooking, be sure to stir the food so that the heat is redistributed and the food cooks evenly.

Cooking times vary slightly, but to give an example, a head of raw broccoli cooks in the microwave in about 6 minutes, depending on the quantity and how soft you like it. A good rule of thumb is to microwave the florets on high for 3 minutes, then check and redistribute them. Cook again in 1-minute intervals until the broccoli is as tender as you like it. Ditto for fresh green beans: cook on high for 2 minutes with a couple of tablespoons of salted water, then shake the container and keep microwaving in 1-minute intervals, checking after each minute.

LEMONY GREEN BEANS IN THE MICROWAVE

In a microwave-safe container or bowl with a cover, microwave 1½ pounds green beans with 3 tablespoons salted water on high for 3 minutes. Shake the container or stir the beans. Replace the cover. Continue to microwave in 1-minute intervals, checking after each minute. Drain when they're tender and bright green, then top with 1 tablespoon freshly squeezed lemon juice. You can heighten the natural flavor of the cooked beans by seasoning them with 1 tablespoon of chopped fresh dill, tarragon, or cilantro or 2 minced shallots that you have cooked briefly in 1 teaspoon melted, reduced-fat, soft tub margarine. Serves 4.

Braising, Poaching, and Roasting

These three cooking methods are good not only for vegetables, but fabulous tasting for meats, fish, and poultry as well.

BRAISING

Most everyone's tasted delicious braised brisket, falling-off-the-bones osso bucco, or a meltingly tender leg of veal. In general, leaner cuts of meat (like brisket, chuck roast, whole turkey breast, and pork chops) take very well to braising. In this method, the food is simmered slowly in liquid in a closed pot, which means it is surrounded by steam. You may use water or another liquid, like wine, beer, or broth. Often, onions, herbs, or garlic are added to flavor the food. By the way, the difference between braising and stewing is that stews contain more liquid and the foods tend to be cut into smaller pieces. For braising, brown the meat in 1 tablespoon of oil before placing it in a baking dish. Add the liquid of your choice until it comes about 1 inch up the sides of the meat. Cover and cook for 2 to 3 hours, depending on the size, either in a low oven (325°) or on top of the stove over medium-low heat.

Denser vegetables, like leeks, carrots, fennel, butternut squash, and potatoes, also take very well to braising.

BRAISED BRISKET WITH ONIONS

Pour 1 tablespoon olive oil into a heavy, ovenproof pan that has a cover. (A Dutch oven works very well.) Place a brisket of beef (about 2½ lbs.) into the pan and brown it on all sides over medium heat. Remove the meat from the pan and season it with 1 teaspoon salt and ¼ teaspoon black pepper. In the same pan, brown 2 cups minced onion in 1 teaspoon of oil. Return the meat to the pan containing the onions. Add 2 cloves of minced garlic, 4 tablespoons tomato paste, and 3 to 4 cups beef broth or water. Cover the pan and braise in a 325° oven for 2 to 3 hours, turning the meat about every half hour, until it's tender. Serves 4 to 6, with leftovers for sandwiches.

BRAISED BROCCOLI

In a heavy pan with a cover, cook 2 cloves of minced garlic in 1 teaspoon olive oil, stirring, over medium-low heat for 2 minutes. Add 1 head broccoli, cut into florets. Stir and cook on medium-low heat for 3 minutes. Pour in 1 cup white wine, cover, and cook for 3 minutes, then continue to cook, uncovered, on medium-low heat until the wine has nearly evaporated, about 5 minutes. Season with salt and freshly ground black pepper to taste. Serves 4 to 6.

POACHING

Poaching is cooking food in a liquid such as stock or water very gently just below the boiling point. Very often, meat and chicken are simmered in broth, and eggs or fish in water. This cooking method, which gives food a very delicate flavor, is easy to do. Following are two popular dishes that employ poaching as a cooking method.

POACHED CHICKEN

In a large soup pot or stockpot, stir together 2½ cups dry white wine, 2½ cups water, 3 sprigs fresh thyme, ½ medium peeled onion, and a celery stalk. Bring to a boil, and add 4 large boneless chicken breasts. Cover and simmer for 20 to 25 minutes. Serves 4.

POACHED SALMON

In a large skillet, combine 1½ cups water, ¼ cup lemon juice, ½ cup sliced onion, 12 whole black peppercorns, 3 sprigs parsley, 1 bay leaf, and ½ teaspoon salt. Bring to a boil and add 6 fresh salmon steaks, each about 1-inch thick. Cover and simmer for 10 minutes or until the fish flakes easily with a fork. Remove the fish from the skillet and discard the liquid. Serve the salmon chilled or hot, garnished with fresh snipped dill or chopped fresh chives. Serves 6.

ROASTING

A dry-heat method best used for more tender meats as well as various vegetables, this involves oven cooking in an uncovered pan. A wonderfully easy method for eggplant, zucchini, onions, cauliflower, broccoli, potatoes, and winter squash, roasting yields vegetables that are browned and crisp on the outside, and sweet and flavorful within. Cut the vegetables into uniformly sized chunks, spray with cooking spray, toss with fresh rosemary, and sprinkle with salt and pepper. Roast in a 425° oven until done, usually about 35 to 40 minutes.

True, this method takes a long time, but the results are well worth it. The longer you cook the vegetables, the more caramelized and tasty they get. It's almost like a decadent vegetable dish you'd expect to find in a four-star French restaurant, where everything is routinely seasoned with cream and gobs of butter. You can make other vegetables in the same way, so prepare plenty in advance. Store in individual plastic containers so you can enjoy them later in the week. Try my easy, very versatile recipe for roasting root vegetables.

ROASTED ROOT VEGETABLES

Place about 6 cups of vegetables (carrots, parsnips, eggplant, turnips, sweet potatoes, onions) in a large bowl. Toss with 1 tablespoon extra-virgin olive oil, 3 or 4 sprigs fresh tarragon, and 6 cloves minced garlic. Sprinkle with 1 teaspoon salt and ½ teaspoon pepper and spread out in a large roasting pan. Roast in a 425° oven for 35 minutes, stirring every 10 minutes. If you like them extra-brown, run them under the oven broiler for 1 minute. Sprinkle with parsley and serve hot or at room temperature. Serves 6.

ROAST CHICKEN

Preheat the oven to 450°. Place 3-pound chicken, trimmed of fat, breast side down, on a rack in a large roasting pan. Stir together 2 tablespoons olive oil, 1 teaspoon chopped fresh thyme, 1 teaspoon chopped fresh rosemary, 1 teaspoon salt, and freshly ground black pepper. Spoon the olive oil mixture over the chicken. Place the chicken in oven and immediately reduce the heat to 325°. Roast, basting every 15 minutes, for about 1 hour. The chicken is done when the thickest part of the thigh reads 165° on a meat thermometer. Allow the chicken to rest for 15 minutes before carving. Discard all the juices that drain off the bird as it rests. Serves 4.

ROAST TURKEY

Preheat the oven to 350°. Place 10- to 12-pound turkey, thawed if frozen, giblets removed and discarded, on a rack in a large roasting pan. Brush the turkey; with 1 tablespoon olive oil. Stuff 1 cup chopped onion; 1 large carrot, peeled and chopped; and 2 stalks celery, peeled and chopped, into the turkey. Pour 1 cup fat-free chicken broth over the turkey. Sprinkle with salt and pepper to taste. Roast, basting every half hour, for 3 to 3½ hours, until an instant-read thermometer inserted into the midthigh reads 165°. Remove the turkey to a platter and allow it to rest for 15 minutes before carving. Serves 8.

Stir-Frying

Crisp, crunchy, and colorful, stir-fried meats and vegetables in a spicy Asian-flavored sauce are irresistible and very versatile; you can toss in whatever ingredients you happen to have on hand. Plus, you need very little or no fat with this cooking method, and the result is so satisfying you'll find yourself turning to stir-fries over and over. Cut up the meat and vegetables into small, even pieces. Then heat 1 tablespoon of oil in a wok or large skillet over medium-high heat until it sizzles when a drop of water hits it. Add the vegetables and meat, and cook quickly, stirring constantly, so that all the surfaces make contact with the heat source. For the liquid, you may use fat-free, low-sodium chicken broth, light teriyaki sauce, or vegetable broth. For two very low-calorie vegetable stir-fries, try the recipes below.

LOW-CAL COLORFUL VEGETABLE STIR-FRY

Cut 1½ pounds broccoli into florets; peel the stalks and cut them into thin strips. Peel, seed, and core 1 red bell pepper and 1 yellow bell pepper and cut into strips. Mince 1 clove garlic. Heat 1 teaspoon peanut oil in a large, nonstick skillet or wok, add all the vegetables, and cook over high heat, stirring, for about 5 minutes. Add ½ teaspoon salt, a pinch of sugar, and 1 cup chicken or beef broth. Cook, stirring, until nearly all the liquid evaporates, about 4 or 5 minutes more. Serves 4 to 6.

STIR-FRY SCALLOPS WITH SNOW PEAS

Spray a large nonstick skillet with cooking spray. Add 1 tablespoon olive oil; 2 cloves garlic, peeled and chopped; and 1½ cups snow peas. Stir-fry over medium heat for about 3 minutes. Add 2 cups sea scallops and stir-fry for 3 to 5 minutes. Sprinkle with salt and pepper to taste. Remove the scallops and snow peas to a bowl. Add the juice of one lemon to the pan and cook over medium-high heat for 1 minute. Return the scallops and snow peas to the skillet and stir to coat with the sauce. Sprinkle with 1 tablespoon parsley. Serves 4.

Sautéing

While recipes for sautéed foods generally call for an overload of butter or oil, this can be a low-fat way to prepare foods if you use a minimum of oil and cook in a nonstick pan sprayed with cooking spray. Some of the plainest vegetables make the most satisfying sautés. For instance, cut plum tomatoes in half and sauté them with minced garlic cloves in 1 teaspoon of olive oil. Season with a splash of balsamic vinegar and sprinkle with salt, freshly ground black pepper, and some chopped fresh basil. Or sauté a chopped onion in ¼ cup of nonfat chicken broth or vegetable juice in a nonstick, covered pan. It takes just minutes, and you'll avoid hundreds of calories by not sautéing these vegetables in loads of oil. Zucchini is wonderful sautéed: slice 3 zucchini into half moons and cook for several minutes in a nonstick pan with 2 cloves minced fresh garlic. Season with 2 teaspoons fresh lemon juice, salt and pepper to taste, and 1 tablespoon chopped fresh dill.

For a nice side dish to roasted meats, prepare an easy "sauté" by cooking a couple of chopped shallots in 1 teaspoon of olive oil for 2 minutes, then adding ½ pound of halved fresh mushrooms. Sauté for 7 minutes or until the mushrooms start to lose their liquid. Season with ½ teaspoon salt, a pinch of freshly ground black pepper, and a pinch of chopped fresh thyme.

SAUTÉED FENNEL AND SAVOY CABBAGE

In a sauté pan, cook 2 minced garlic cloves in 1 teaspoon olive oil for 1 minute, then add 1 thinly sliced head of savoy cabbage and 1 thinly sliced fennel bulb. Cook for 3 minutes, just till crisp. Stir in a pinch of fennel seed and season to taste with salt and pepper. Serves 4 to 6.

Measurements, Substitutions, and Such

If you don't have a particular ingredient for a dish you are making, don't panic! No matter what you're making, you can always substitute something. Here is a list of substitutes.

Baking powder (1 teaspoon)　Substitute ½ teaspoon cream of tartar and ¼ teaspoon baking soda.

Beef or chicken broth (1 cup)   Substitute 1 teaspoon instant beef or chicken bouillon plus 1 cup water.

Breadcrumbs, dry (½ cup)   Substitute ½ cup cornflake crumbs or ½ cup cracker crumbs.

Buttermilk (1 cup)   Substitute 1 tablespoon lemon juice or vinegar and enough milk to measure 1 cup, or 1 cup plain yogurt.

Chocolate, semisweet (1 ounce square)   Substitute 3 tablespoons semisweet chocolate pieces or 1 ounce unsweetened chocolate plus 1 tablespoon granulated sugar.

Egg (1)   Substitute 2 egg whites or ¼ cup liquid egg substitute.

Flour, cake (1 cup)   Substitute 1 cup minus 2 tablespoons all-purpose flour.

Flour, self-rising (1 cup)   Substitute 1 cup all-purpose flour mixed with 1 teaspoon baking powder, ½ teaspoon salt, and ¼ teaspoon baking soda.

Garlic (1 clove)   Substitute ⅛ teaspoon garlic powder.

Ginger, freshly grated (1 teaspoon)   Substitute ¼ teaspoon powdered ground ginger.

Herbs, fresh (1 tablespoon)   Substitute 1 teaspoon dried herbs.

Lemon juice (1 teaspoon)   Substitute ½ teaspoon vinegar.

Milk, skim (1 cup)   Substitute ½ cup evaporated skim milk and ½ cup water, or 1 cup water plus ⅓ cup nonfat dry milk powder.

Mushrooms (½ pound fresh)   Substitute 6-ounce can, drained.

Onion, chopped (1 small)   Substitute 1 teaspoon onion powder.

Sour cream (1 cup)   Substitute 1 cup nonfat plain yogurt.

Tomato juice (1 cup)   Substitute ½ cup tomato sauce and ½ cup water.

Tomato sauce (2 cups)   Substitute ¾ cup tomato paste and 1 cup water.

Equivalents

Not sure how many potatoes equal a pound? Unsure how many graham crackers equals a cup of crumbs? Read on for at-a-glance equivalents.

Apples	=	1 pound fresh equals 3 medium apples or 3 cups of sliced apples.
Asparagus	=	1 pound equals 16 to 20 stalks.
Bananas	=	1 medium equals 1 cup sliced.
Beans, black	=	1 pound dried equals 4½ cups cooked.
Beans, green	=	1 pound fresh equals 3½ cups whole.
Blueberries	=	1 pint equals 2 cups.
Broccoli	=	1 pound fresh equals 2 cups chopped.
Cabbage	=	1 pound equals 3½ cups shredded or 2 cups cooked.
Cantaloupe	=	1 medium equals 3 cups diced.
Carrots	=	1 pound equals 3 cups chopped or 2 cups cooked.
Cauliflower	=	1 pound equals 1¾ cups florets.
Celery	=	2 medium-sized ribs equal ½ cup chopped.
Cheese, cheddar	=	½ pound equals 2 cups shredded.
Cheese, cottage	=	16 ounces equal 2 cups.
Cherries	=	1 pound fresh equals 2½ cups pitted.
Chicken, breast	=	1 large equals 1½ cups cooked meat.
Chicken, whole	=	3 pounds equal 3 cups cooked.
Chocolate chips	=	6 ounces equal 1 cup.
Corn	=	2 medium ears equal 1½ cups kernels.
Couscous	=	1 cup uncooked equals 2½ cups cooked.
Crumbs, graham crackers	=	21 squares equal 1½ cups.
Crumbs, vanilla wafer	=	38 cookies equal 1½ cups.
Crumbs, saltine	=	29 wafers equal 1 cup.
Cucumber	=	¾ medium equals 1 cup chopped.
Eggplant	=	1 pound equals 1¾ cups cooked.
Egg whites	=	1 dozen large equals 1½ cups.
Egg yolks	=	1 dozen large equals ⅞ cup.

Eggs, hard-boiled	=	1 egg equals ½ cup chopped.
Eggs, whole	=	1 dozen large equals 2⅓ cups.
Flour	=	1 pound equals 3½ cups.
Garlic	=	1 head equals 12 to 16 cloves.
Grapefruit	=	1 pound equals 1½ cups segments.
Grapes	=	1 pound equals 2½ cups.
Herbs	=	1 tablespoon fresh chopped equals 1 teaspoon dried chopped.
Lemons	=	1 pound equals about 5 medium.
Lentils	=	1 pound dried equals 4 cups cooked.
Lettuce	=	1 pound equals 6 cups pieces.
Mango	=	1 medium equals ¾ cup chopped.
Milk	=	1 quart equals 4 cups.
Mushrooms	=	1 pound equals 6 cups sliced.
Mustard	=	1 teaspoon dry equals 1 tablespoon prepared.
Nectarines	=	1 pound equals 3 medium.
Oats, rolled	=	1 pound equals 5 cups uncooked.
Onions	=	1 pound equals 4 medium or 4 cups chopped.
Oranges	=	1 pound equals 3 medium.
Papaya	=	1 medium equals 1½ cups sliced.
Peaches	=	1 pound equals 4 medium or 2 cups sliced.
Pears	=	1 pound equals 3 medium or 2 cups sliced.
Peas, green	=	1 pound fresh in the pod equals 1 cup shelled.
Peppers, bell	=	1 pound equals 2 large or 2 cups chopped.
Pineapple	=	1 medium equals 4 cups cubed.
Plums	=	1 pound equals 2½ cups sliced or 2 cups cooked.
Potatoes, sweet	=	1 pound equals 3 medium.
Potatoes, white or red	=	1 pound equals 4 cups sliced or 2 cups mashed.
Raspberries	=	½ pint equals 1¼ cups.
Rhubarb	=	1 pound equals 2 cups cooked.
Rice	=	1 cup uncooked equals 3 cups cooked.
Scallops	=	1 pound medium equals 2 cups.
Spinach	=	1 pound fresh equals 10 cups or 1½ cups cooked.

Squash, summer	=	1 pound equals 3 medium or 3 cups sliced.
Squash, winter	=	1 pound equals 1 cup cooked, mashed.
Strawberries	=	1 pint equals 1½ cups sliced.
Tangerines	=	1 pound equals 4 medium.
Tomato paste	=	6-ounce can equals ¾ cup.
Tomatoes	=	1 pound equals 3 medium or 2 cups sliced.
Tuna	=	6-ounce can equals ⅔ cup drained.
Turkey	=	12-pound bird equals 15 to 16 cups cooked meat.

My Top Ten Tips for Getting the Most Flavor from the Foods You Eat

In a myriad of wonderful, remarkably simple ways, you can boost the flavor in the foods you eat without adding much in the way of calories.

1. **Know your ingredients.** Sure, cheese is high in fat, but you can maximize the flavor by using a small amount of a strongly flavored type, like feta or blue cheese, rather than a lot of a mild cheese like Muenster.

2. **Substitute lower-calorie dairy products.** Use buttermilk in place of sour cream—it's low in fat and calories and has a lot of the creaminess and flavor of sour cream. Use evaporated skim milk in place of cream in sauces and thicken the sauce with a bit of flour or cornstarch as needed. For instance, Pretty in Pink Strawberry Soup uses evaporated fat-free milk in place of cream for a silken, luxuriously thick texture and pure flavor. And Slow-Cooker Beef Stroganoff substitutes light sour cream for regular sour cream, thus eliminating hundreds of calories without sacrificing taste.

3. **Whenever you substitute, use an equivalent amount.** For instance, if your pumpkin pie recipe calls for 1 cup of heavy cream, substitute 1 cup of evaporated skim milk.

4. **Rethink how you cook chicken.** For a juicier, less fatty, more flavorful bird, stick a handful of fresh herbs underneath the skin of the poultry before cooking. The meat will be deliciously infused with the flavor of thyme, tarragon, or marjoram. Removing the skin from

poultry saves you plenty of fat calories, but do so after the cooking, not before. (The meat won't absorb much fat during the cooking and the flavorful seasoning will remain underneath.)

5. Choose Canadian-style, turkey, or soy bacon. These all have substantially fewer calories than regular bacon but just as much flavor. And instead of pork sausage, look for extra-lean chicken, turkey, or soy sausage.

6. Nuts lend crunch, texture, and taste. They also add a lot of calories, but just a small amount can enhance a meal: garnish stir-fried broccoli for four with 1 tablespoon chopped walnuts and you've added just 18 calories per serving. To enhance their flavor, always toast nuts before using.

7. Puree mashed potatoes with reduced-sodium chicken broth or the cooking liquid. Omit the butter, or add just 1 tablespoon. You can boost both the flavor and the nutritional content and decrease the calorie content of mashed potatoes by using half pureed cauliflower and half potatoes.

8. Replace fat. When making an otherwise calorie-laden sauce such as pesto or garlic and olive oil for pasta, save a little bit of the cooking water when you boil the noodles. Replace half the fat in the recipe with cooking water, and you'll save hundreds of calories.

9. Use cooking spray instead of butter or oil to grease pans as well as to sauté meat and vegetables. You'll save unnecessary calories.

10. Make your food look fabulous. Whether you're eating a piece of grilled fish or a stew, pay attention to how it looks. Food that looks good always tastes better. Think visually! If you're having chicken breast, serve it with a colorful vegetable like broccoli or carrots rather than cauliflower, which is the same color. If you make a low-fat onion dip with fat-free sour cream, spoon it into a hollowed-out green, yellow, or red bell pepper and sprinkle the top with some chopped scallion. Shepherd's Pie with Turkey and Cauliflower looks bright and appetizing when you arrange thin slices of red pepper across the top for color. Stuff tuna or egg salad (made with low-fat mayonnaise) into a hollowed-out bell pepper or tomato. Grate some baby carrots and sprinkle over salads and soups. Fruit salads look more festive when you garnish them with strips of orange peel or mint leaves. When you serve fish, decorate the plate with a lime or lemon twist. Simply cut a slice from the fruit and twist in opposite directions. A simple salad looks more appetizing when decorated with tomato slices that you have dipped into chopped fresh parsley.

Now that you've mastered my smart shopping strategies and kitchen techniques, you're ready to cook. By now, you're prepared to whip up energizing breakfasts, delicious lunches that will make you feel satisfied, and fabulous dinners that the whole family will enjoy. A whole chapter of gourmet meal ideas, another one on preparing healthy meals kids love, plus a large batch of fun foods will give you everything you need to eat well and lose weight. Let's get started!

Part II   Cooking with Joy!

Four

Breakfast: Recipes to Break the Fast

This chapter offers a variety of energizing breakfasts that will help get your day off to a great start. They're easy enough to make for yourself and delicious enough to serve to your family, friends, and morning guests.

If you're following the 1,200-calorie a day plan, you'll notice that each breakfast has been portioned out to provide your allotted 200-calorie amount. For those following the 1,400- or the

1,600-calorie plan, you'll be eating about 250 calories at breakfast. For the 1,800-calorie participants, breakfast portions total 300 calories. And for those of you who are superactive, maintaining your weight, or simply looking for great, healthy breakfast ideas, the 2,000-calorie plan portions are 350 calories. Simply check underneath the recipe and find the portion instructions (and food accompaniments) for your personal caloric level. The math has already been done, so all you'll need to do is enjoy the food. Also, you may drink unlimited plain coffee or tea, though if you are caffeine sensitive, you'll want to limit your consumption.

Because every breakfast has been perfectly manipulated to provide ample nutrition and meet your personal 90/10 plan, you may want to eat a particular meal every day. That's fine. However, variety is the key to staying satisfied, so don't automatically limit yourself to just one dish.

If you love carbs first thing in the morning, try Cranberry Pecan Scones or the bursting-with-fruit Oatmeal Berry Muffins. Either is great to savor on the weekend when you're lounging with the newspaper. Trying to bump up your calcium intake? Sample Blueberry Yogurt Pancakes, with 190 milligrams of calcium per serving, or Fruity Tofu Yogurt Shake, with 302 milligrams of calcium in a serving. And if you prefer a protein-rich meal to start the day, the Cheddar Mushroom Omelet's got 21 grams of protein to give you plenty of staying power. So browse through this incredibly varied collection of breakfast recipes—you're sure to find some that will become personal favorites!

Apple Cinnamon Crepes

Serves 6 (2 crepes each)

Tender crepes envelop a flavorful fruit filling that's gently spiced with maple syrup and cinnamon for a breakfast that will make you feel like a pampered Parisian.

CREPES
⅔ cup all-purpose flour
½ teaspoon cinnamon
⅔ cup skim milk
1 tablespoon vegetable oil
3 egg whites
Vegetable oil spray

FILLING
Vegetable oil spray
3 Granny Smith apples, peeled, cored, and chopped
1 teaspoon brown sugar
Pinch of cinnamon
1 tablespoon reduced-sugar maple syrup
Juice of ½ lemon
¼ teaspoon vanilla extract

1. Make the crepes: In a medium mixing bowl, stir together the flour and cinnamon. Add the milk, oil, and egg whites. Beat well. Cover and refrigerate for 1 to 3 hours.

2. Spray a nonstick crepe pan or a 6- to 7-inch sauté pan with vegetable oil spray. Heat over medium heat until the pan is hot. Add about 2 tablespoons batter to the pan and tilt the pan to distribute the batter evenly across the bottom. Return the pan to the heat and cook the crepe until golden brown. Flip the crepe over and cook the other side for 30 seconds. Place crepes on a plate and allow to cool.

3. Make the filling: Spray an 8- or 10-inch nonstick sauté pan with vegetable oil spray. Add the apples and sauté for 8 to 10 minutes, until soft. Add the brown sugar and cinnamon. Stir in the syrup and cook 1 minute. Remove from the heat and stir in the lemon juice and vanilla.

4. Spoon 2 tablespoons apple mixture into center of each crepe. Roll the crepes around the filling. Place the crepes, seam side down, on a serving plate. Serve warm.

NUTRIENT ANALYSIS

◆ 1 SERVING = 2 CREPES

Calories: 135	Protein: 4.3 g	Carbohydrates: 24 g	Sugar: 11 g	Total fat: 2.7 g
Saturated fat: 0 g	Cholesterol: 0 g	Sodium: 46 mg	Fiber: 2.7 g	Calcium: 49 mg

1,200-CALORIE PLAN

1 serving crepes
1/2 cup nonfat vanilla yogurt

1,400- & 1,600-CALORIE PLANS

1 serving crepes
1 cup nonfat vanilla yogurt

1,800-CALORIE PLAN

1 1/2 servings crepes
1/2 cup nonfat vanilla yogurt
1 tablespoon low-fat granola cereal

2,000-CALORIE PLAN

1 1/2 servings crepes
1 cup nonfat vanilla yogurt
1 tablespoon low-fat granola cereal

Blueberry Yogurt Pancakes

Serves 4 (2 pancakes each)

These light-as-a-cloud pancakes, bursting with ripe berries, are just what you'd expect to find at a bed-and-breakfast in Maine. They're also extremely easy to make since all the ingredients get whipped up in a blender.

1 egg
1 cup plain, nonfat yogurt
1 tablespoon canola oil
1 cup all-purpose flour
1 tablespoon sugar
1 teaspoon baking powder
$\frac{1}{2}$ teaspoon baking soda
Pinch of salt
$\frac{1}{4}$ teaspoon cinnamon
$\frac{1}{2}$ cup fresh or frozen blueberries

1. In a blender, combine the egg, yogurt, and oil. Blend until smooth.

2. Sift together the flour, sugar, baking powder, baking soda, salt, and cinnamon. Add to the yogurt mixture and blend well.

3. Spray a hot griddle with cooking spray. Using about $\frac{1}{8}$ of the batter for each pancake, ladle the pancakes onto the griddle. Sprinkle each with some blueberries and cook for about 30 seconds (or until bubbles form in the middle of pancake). Flip over and cook until golden.

NUTRIENT ANALYSIS

◆ 1 SERVING = 2 PANCAKES

Calories: 219	Protein: 8.5 g	Carbohydrates: 35 g	Sugar: 7.8 g	Total fat: 5 g
Saturated fat: 0.75 g	Cholesterol: 54 mg	Sodium: 295 mg	Fiber: 1.5 g	Calcium: 19 mg

1,200-CALORIE PLAN

1 serving pancakes

1,400- & 1,600-CALORIE PLANS

1 serving pancakes

2 tablespoons low-fat sour cream

1,800-CALORIE PLAN

1 serving pancakes

2 tablespoons low-fat sour cream

2 teaspoons slivered almonds

2,000-CALORIE PLAN

1 serving pancakes

2 tablespoons low-fat sour cream

2 tablespoons slivered almonds

Grandma's Cheese Pancakes

Serves 3 (4 pancakes each)

You'd never know that these tender, thin flapjacks were made with cottage cheese (don't tell your kids!). With 18 grams of protein per serving, these keep you feeling satisfied for hours, and they're incredibly easy to make.

2 eggs, whole
1 egg white
1¼ cups 1% low-fat cottage cheese
1 tablespoon reduced-fat, soft tub margarine
⅓ cup all-purpose flour
1 tablespoon Splenda (or 1 tablespoon granulated white sugar)

1. In a food processor or by hand, beat the eggs and egg white for 20 seconds. Add the remaining ingredients and mix until smooth. Allow the batter to rest for 10 to 15 minutes.

2. Spray large, nonstick skillet with cooking spray and heat over a medium flame until very hot. Spoon 1 heaping tablespoon of batter per pancake onto the skillet and cook over medium heat, about 1 minute on each side, until golden.

NUTRIENT ANALYSIS

◆ **1 SERVING = 4 PANCAKES**

Calories: 157	Protein: 18 g	Carbohydrates: 14 g	Sugar: 2.7 g	Total fat: 4.4 g
Saturated fat: 1.6 g	Cholesterol: 145 mg	Sodium: 473 mg	Fiber: 0.3 g	Calcium: 86 mg

1,200-CALORIE PLAN

1 serving pancakes
$\frac{1}{4}$ cantaloupe or $\frac{1}{2}$ cup blueberries

1,400- & 1,600-CALORIE PLANS

1 serving pancakes
$\frac{1}{2}$ cantaloupe or 1 cup blueberries

1,800-CALORIE PLAN

1$\frac{1}{2}$ servings pancakes (6 pancakes)
$\frac{1}{4}$ cantaloupe or $\frac{1}{2}$ cup blueberries

2,000-CALORIE PLAN

2 servings pancakes (8 pancakes)
$\frac{1}{4}$ cantaloupe or $\frac{1}{2}$ cup blueberries

Pineapple Cheese Pancakes

Serves 3 (5 small pancakes each)

If you like pineapple cheesecake, try these guilt-free, decadent pancakes. They're great to make for a leisurely weekend breakfast when the whole family is in the mood for something special.

2 eggs, whole
1 egg white
1½ cups 1% low-fat cottage cheese
1 tablespoon reduced-fat, soft tub margarine
⅓ cup all-purpose flour
1 tablespoon Splenda (or 1 tablespoon granulated white sugar)
5 heaping tablespoons crushed, canned pineapple, fully drained

1. In a food processor or by hand, beat the eggs and egg white for 20 seconds. Add the cottage cheese, margarine, flour, and Splenda. Mix well.

2. In a bowl, combine the batter and the pineapple. Mix thoroughly and allow the batter to rest for 10 to 15 minutes.

3. Spray a large, nonstick skillet with cooking spray and heat over a medium flame until very hot. Spoon 1 heaping tablespoon of batter per pancake onto the skillet and cook over medium heat. Gently press down on the pancakes with a spatula to flatten. Flip and brown both sides evenly. Remove the cakes when they are firm and golden.

NUTRIENT ANALYSIS				
◆ 1 SERVING = 5 PANCAKES				
Calories: 204	Protein: 20 g	Carbohydrates: 18 g	Sugar: 7.7 g	Total fat: 4.6 g
Saturated fat: 1.7 g	Cholesterol: 147 mg	Sodium: 550 mg	Fiber: 0.6 g	Calcium: 102 mg

1,200-CALORIE PLAN

1 serving pancakes

1,400- & 1,600-CALORIE PLANS

1 serving pancakes
$1/2$ cup fresh pineapple, cubed

1,800-CALORIE PLAN

1 serving pancakes
1 cup fresh pineapple, cubed

2,000-CALORIE PLAN

$1^{1}/2$ servings pancakes ($7^{1}/2$ pancakes)
$1/2$ cup fresh pineapple, cubed

Strawberry Oat Pancakes

Serves 6 (2 pancakes each)

A topping of sliced strawberries is prettier and lighter than regular pancake syrup, and just as satisfying. Be sure to buy the ripest berries you can find. You can substitute fresh raspberries.

1 cup all-purpose flour
½ cup quick-cooking rolled oats, uncooked
1 tablespoon baking powder
2 tablespoons Splenda
½ teaspoon salt
1 cup skim milk
1 egg (or ¼ cup egg substitute)
2 tablespoons vegetable oil
1 cup sliced fresh strawberries

1. Heat a large griddle over medium-high heat or preheat an electric griddle to 375°.

2. In a large mixing bowl, stir together the flour, oats, baking powder, Splenda, and salt.

3. In another bowl, vigorously whisk together the milk, egg, and oil.

4. Combine the liquid and dry ingredients, and stir just until the dry ingredients are moistened.

5. Form 12 pancakes on the griddle. Use 1 heaping tablespoon of batter per pancake. Cook on one side until the tops are covered with bubbles and the edges look dry. Turn over and cook until done.

6. Garnish with the sliced strawberries.

◆ **1 SERVING = 2 PANCAKES**

Calories: 216	Protein: 6 g	Carbohydrates: 35 g	Sugar: 13 g	Total fat: 6 g
Saturated fat: 0.8 g	Cholesterol: 0 mg	Sodium: 236 mg	Fiber: 2 g	Calcium: 180 mg

1,200-CALORIE PLAN

1 serving pancakes

1,400- & 1,600-CALORIE PLANS

1 serving pancakes
2 soy breakfast links

1,800-CALORIE PLAN

1 serving pancakes
3 soy breakfast links

2,000-CALORIE PLAN

1 serving pancakes
2 soy breakfast links
1 egg, hard-boiled, poached, or scrambled in
cooking spray

Cottage Cheese Rice Bowls

Serves 12

Try these healthful minicasseroles when you've got leftover brown rice. They're savory and satisfying—and especially nice to serve for brunch since each batch makes a bunch. You can replace the cottage cheese with nonfat flavored yogurt or unsweetened applesauce.

3 cups cooked brown rice
⅓ cup soy milk or skim milk
1 cup shredded low-fat cheddar cheese
½ cup chopped frozen spinach, cooked and drained
2 eggs, beaten
½ teaspoon salt
½ teaspoon freshly ground black pepper
2 cups 1% low-fat cottage cheese

1. Preheat the oven to 400°.

2. Combine all the ingredients except the cottage cheese and mix thoroughly.

3. Evenly divide the mixture into a 12-cup muffin tin coated with cooking spray or lined with muffin cups.

4. Bake for 20 minutes (or until set). Let the rice bowls cool slightly and scoop in 1 heaping tablespoon of cottage cheese.

NUTRIENT ANALYSIS

♦ **1 SERVING = 1 COTTAGE CHEESE RICE BOWL**

Calories: 146	Protein: 12 g	Carbohydrates: 13.7 g	Sugar: 1.5 g	Total fat: 5 g
Saturated fat: 2.5 g	Cholesterol: 50 mg	Sodium: 332 mg	Fiber: 1.3 g	Calcium: 189 mg

1,200-CALORIE PLAN

1 rice bowl

$1/2$ grapefruit or 1 orange

1,400- & 1,600-CALORIE PLANS

1 rice bowl

1 sliced banana or 1 cup blueberries

1,800-CALORIE PLAN

1 rice bowl

1 sliced banana and $1/4$ cubed cantaloupe

2,000-CALORIE PLAN

2 rice bowls

$1/2$ grapefruit or 1 orange

Cheddar Mushroom Omelet

Serves 1

Make this country-style omelet when you're in the mood for a filling, hearty breakfast. It'll remind you of the hefty omelets served at the local diner—but with a fraction of the fat and calories. If you're pressed for time, you can sauté the mushrooms and dice the cheese the night before and refrigerate them, tightly covered, until you're ready to cook.

Vegetable oil cooking spray
6 large mushrooms, thinly sliced
1 egg
2 egg whites
1 small slice reduced-fat cheddar cheese, diced
Parsley sprigs, for garnish

1. Spray the bottom of an 8- or 10-inch nonstick sauté pan with cooking spray. Over medium heat, sauté the mushrooms for 3 to 4 minutes, until softened.

2. In a small bowl, beat the egg with the egg whites until foamy. Pour the eggs over the mushrooms. Sprinkle the cheese on top. Cook the omelet over medium heat, tilting the pan to allow the uncooked portion of egg to run out to the edges of the pan as you pull the cooked portion toward the center of the pan with a spatula.

3. When the omelet is fairly firm, fold it over in half and cook 1 or 2 minutes longer, pressing down on it with a spatula. Flip to cook and brown the underside.

4. When there is no trace of uncooked egg remaining, remove the omelet from the pan to a plate. Garnish with parsley sprigs.

NUTRIENT ANALYSIS				
Calories: 169	Protein: 21 g	Carbohydrates: 7.5 g	Sugar: 4.1 g	Total fat: 7 g
Saturated fat: 1.8 g	Cholesterol: 215 mg	Sodium: 449 mg	Fiber: 1 g	Calcium: 186 mg

1,200-CALORIE PLAN

1 omelet

1 slice 40-calorie whole wheat bread, toasted

1,400- & 1,600-CALORIE PLANS

1 omelet

2 slices 40-calorie whole wheat bread, toasted

1,800-CALORIE PLAN

1 omelet

2 slices 40-calorie whole wheat bread, toasted

2 veggie breakfast links

2,000-CALORIE PLAN

1 omelet

2 slices 40-calorie whole wheat bread, toasted

1 tablespoon reduced-fat, soft-tub margarine

2 veggie breakfast links

Vegetable Frittata

Serves 4

Loads of colorful, crunchy garden vegetables fill this egg dish, which gets a lively flavor from the fresh basil. A run under the oven broiler after cooking ensures a golden brown topping.

Vegetable oil cooking spray
1 cup broccoli florets
1 cup diced red pepper
1 cup diced yellow pepper
1 cup diced green pepper
1 cup thinly sliced zucchini
1 cup thinly sliced mushrooms
½ cup chopped onion
3 eggs
5 egg whites
½ cup 1% low-fat cottage cheese
¼ cup chopped fresh basil
½ teaspoon freshly ground black pepper
4 tablespoons freshly grated Parmesan cheese

1. Preheat the oven broiler.

2. Generously spray a 10-inch ovenproof skillet with cooking spray. In the skillet, sauté all the vegetables for 4 to 5 minutes, until crisp-tender.

3. Meanwhile, in a mixing bowl, combine the eggs and egg whites. Beat thoroughly with a whisk. Mix in the cottage cheese, basil, and pepper.

4. Pour the egg mixture over the sautéed vegetables in the skillet. Cook, uncovered, for several minutes, until the frittata is firm and golden brown on the bottom. As the frittata cooks, lift up the sides occasionally with a spatula and tilt the pan so that the uncooked egg runs underneath and cooks. Remove the skillet from the heat.

5. Sprinkle the top of the frittata evenly with the Parmesan cheese. Place the skillet under the oven broiler, about 5 inches from the heat. Broil for 2 minutes, until the top is golden brown.

6. Cut into 4 wedges.

NUTRIENT ANALYSIS

♦ **1 SERVING = ¼ OF FRITTATA**

Calories: 190	Protein: 18.6 g	Carbohydrates: 15.8 g	Sugar: 5 g	Total fat: 6.3 g
Saturated fat: 2.4 g	Cholesterol: 164 mg	Sodium: 342 mg	Fiber: 4.3 g	Calcium: 147 mg

1,200-CALORIE PLAN

1 serving frittata

1,400- & 1,600-CALORIE PLANS

1 serving frittata
1 slice 40-calorie whole wheat bread, toasted
1 teaspoon reduced-fat, soft tub margarine

1,800-CALORIE PLAN

1 serving frittata
2 slices 40-calorie whole wheat bread, toasted
1 teaspoon reduced-fat, soft tub margarine

2,000-CALORIE PLAN

1½ serving frittata
1 slice 40-calorie whole wheat bread, toasted
1 teaspoon reduced-fat, soft tub margarine

Scrambled Egg Whites, Lox, and Tomato

Serves 1

My Sunday morning special is both delicious and filling because it's made with three egg whites in addition to a whole egg. Try doubling the recipe and making it for someone special on a weekend morning. Serve on warmed plates, and set the table with fresh flowers.

Cooking spray
¼ onion, chopped
2 ounces lox, cut into small pieces
1 whole egg, beaten
3 egg whites, beaten
¼ tomato, chopped
Salt and freshly ground black pepper

1. Coat a skillet with cooking spray and sauté the onions until soft and slightly browned.

2. Add the lox, egg, and egg whites, and gently scramble. Be sure to cook just until the eggs are set.

3. Add the chopped tomatoes and salt and pepper.

NUTRIENT ANALYSIS				
Calories: 207	Protein: 28 g	Carbohydrates: 5.4 g	Sugar: 1.5 g	Total fat: 7.6 g
Saturated fat: 2 g	Cholesterol: 225 mg	Sodium: 1364 mg	Fiber: 1 g	Calcium: 44 mg

1,200-CALORIE PLAN

1 serving scrambled eggs

1,400- & 1,600-CALORIE PLANS

1 serving scrambled eggs
1 slice 40-calorie whole wheat bread, toasted

1,800-CALORIE PLAN

1 serving scrambled eggs
2 slices 40-calorie whole wheat bread, toasted

2,000-CALORIE PLAN

1 serving scrambled eggs
2 slices 40-calorie whole wheat bread, toasted
1 tablespoon reduced-fat, soft tub margarine or cream cheese

Applesauce Muffins

Makes 12

You get a double hit of fruit flavor in these lightly spiced muffins, thanks to both applesauce and chopped fresh apple. They're best served warm right from the oven, though you can also freeze them, tightly wrapped, for up to three months.

2¼ cups all-purpose flour
1¼ cups sugar (or Splenda)
1 teaspoon baking soda
1 teaspoon baking powder
1 teaspoon salt
2 teaspoons ground cinnamon
1⅓ cups natural, unsweetened applesauce
⅓ cup canola oil
2 whole eggs, lightly beaten
1 medium apple, peeled and chopped

1. Preheat the oven to 350°. Spray a 12-cup nonstick muffin tin with vegetable oil spray.

2. In a large bowl, sift together the flour, sugar, baking soda, baking powder, salt, and cinnamon. Mix in the applesauce, oil, and eggs. Blend at low speed until moistened, then beat another 2 minutes on high speed. Stir in the chopped apple.

3. Pour the batter into the muffin tin and bake for 18 to 20 minutes. Remove from tin and allow muffins to cool slightly.

NUTRIENT ANALYSIS

◆ **1 SERVING = 1 MUFFIN**

Calories: 198	Protein: 3.5 g	Carbohydrates: 30 g	Sugar: 10 g	Total fat: 7 g
Saturated fat: 0.7 g	Cholesterol: 35 mg	Sodium: 311 mg	Fiber: 1.2 g	Calcium: 61 mg

1,200-CALORIE PLAN

1 muffin

1,400- & 1,600-CALORIE PLANS

1 muffin
$1/2$ cup blueberries or $1/4$ cantaloupe

1,800-CALORIE PLAN

1 muffin
$1/2$ cup nonfat flavored yogurt or $1/4$ cup 1
  percent low-fat cottage cheese
$1/2$ cup blueberries or $1/4$ cantaloupe

2,000-CALORIE PLAN

1 muffin
1 cup nonfat flavored yogurt or $1/2$ cup 1
  percent low-fat cottage cheese
$1/2$ cup blueberries or $1/4$ cantaloupe

Oatmeal Berry Muffins

Makes 12

If you measure out the dry ingredients the night before, it takes just a few minutes in the morning to assemble the batter for these fruit- and nut-filled gems. The mouthwatering aroma as they bake will motivate all sleepyheads to wake up and get moving. Also, the oats provide soluble fiber—the type that helps stabilize your blood sugar. Store at room temperature for 1 to 2 days, or freeze for up to three months.

1 cup all-purpose flour
1 cup uncooked old-fashioned oats
¼ cup packed brown sugar
½ cup ground flaxseeds
1 teaspoon baking powder
1 teaspoon baking soda
¼ teaspoon salt
1 teaspoon cinnamon
8 ounces nonfat vanilla yogurt
2 egg whites, beaten
1 tablespoon canola oil
1 teaspoon vanilla extract
1 cup fresh or frozen blueberries
1 tablespoon Splenda
1 tablespoon chopped walnuts

1. Preheat the oven to 400°. Spray 12 muffin cups with cooking spray.

2. In a large bowl, combine the flour, oats, brown sugar, flaxseeds, baking powder, baking soda, salt, and ½ teaspoon cinnamon.

3. In a separate bowl, combine the yogurt, egg whites, canola oil, and vanilla. Slowly stir into flour-oat mixture and mix until well blended.

4. Fold in the blueberries, then spoon the entire mixture evenly into the 12 muffin cups.

5. Mix the Splenda, remaining ½ teaspoon cinnamon, and chopped walnuts. Sprinkle over the muffin mixture.

6. Bake for 18 to 20 minutes or until lightly browned. Muffins are done when an inserted toothpick comes out clean.

NUTRIENT ANALYSIS

◆ **1 SERVING = 1 MUFFIN**

Calories: 163	Protein: 5.4 g	Carbohydrates: 26 g	Sugar: 8.3 g	Total fat: 4.5 g
Saturated fat: 0.5 g	Cholesterol: 0 g	Sodium: 186 mg	Fiber: 3 g	Calcium: 95 mg

1,200-CALORIE PLAN

1 muffin
½ grapefruit

1,400- & 1,600-CALORIE PLANS

1 muffin
1 egg, hard-boiled, or scrambled using cooking spray

1,800-CALORIE PLAN

1 muffin
1 egg, hard-boiled, or scrambled using cooking spray
½ grapefruit

2,000-CALORIE PLAN

1 muffin
1 egg + 2 egg whites, hard-boiled, or scrambled using cooking spray
1 apple or 1 cup fresh pineapple chunks

Pumpkin Muffins

Makes 12

The grated orange peel highlights the pumpkin flavor in these fine breakfast muffins, which are just sweet enough that you'll feel almost like you're eating a cupcake. You can freeze the muffins, tightly wrapped, for up to three months.

Cooking spray
½ cup brown sugar
1½ cups whole wheat flour
2 teaspoons baking powder
1 teaspoon cinnamon
½ teaspoon salt
1 egg
1 cup fat-free milk
½ cup canned pumpkin
¼ cup oil
½ teaspoon grated orange peel

1. Preheat the oven to 375°. Lightly spray 12 muffin cups with cooking spray.

2. In a large mixing bowl, stir together the brown sugar, flour, baking powder, cinnamon, and salt.

3. In a separate bowl, beat the egg for 30 seconds or until foamy. Add the milk, pumpkin, oil, and orange peel. Beat well. Add the egg mixture to the flour mixture and stir until the flour mixture is moistened.

4. Spoon the batter into the muffin cups, filling them about three-quarters full. Bake for 15 minutes or until the tops spring back when you press them lightly with a finger. Remove the muffins from the pans and cool on a wire rack.

NUTRIENT ANALYSIS

◆ **1 SERVING = 1 MUFFIN**

Calories: 131	Protein: 3.4 g	Carbohydrates: 19 g	Sugar: 6.9 g	Total fat: 5.3 g
Saturated fat: 0 g	Cholesterol: 18 mg	Sodium: 20 mg	Fiber: 2.3 g	Calcium: 78 mg
Potassium: 226 mg	Vitamin A: 2319 IU			

1,200-CALORIE PLAN

1 muffin
2 tablespoons raw almonds, toasted

1,400- & 1,600-CALORIE PLANS

1 muffin
3 tablespoons raw almonds, toasted

1,800-CALORIE PLAN

1 muffin
4 tablespoons raw almonds, toasted

2,000-CALORIE PLAN

1 muffin
5 tablespoons raw almonds, toasted

Cranberry Pecan Scones

Serves 6

Scones have gotten so popular that most of the doughnut and coffee chains now sell them. Although scones are typically loaded with fat, this version is bursting with fruit and nut flavor thanks to the fresh cranberries and pecans. You can freeze them, tightly wrapped, for up to three months.

1 cup fresh cranberries
2 tablespoons water
¼ cup Splenda
2 cups all-purpose flour
2 teaspoons baking powder
½ teaspoon baking soda
½ teaspoon salt
2 tablespoons reduced-fat, soft tub margarine
1 egg white
¾ cup buttermilk
¼ cup whole pecans, chopped

1. Preheat the oven to 400°. Coat a baking sheet with cooking spray.

2. Pour the cranberries into a small saucepan. Add the water and half the Splenda (⅛ cup), and heat over a medium flame, stirring constantly. The mixture will begin to thicken and the cranberries will melt into a chunky sauce. This will take at least 10 minutes. Cover and set aside.

3. In a large mixing bowl, combine the flour, remaining Splenda, baking powder, baking soda, and salt. Thoroughly mix. Add the margarine and continue to mix.

4. In a small bowl, combine the egg white and buttermilk. Add to the flour mixture.

5. Lightly dust your work surface with flour (to prevent the dough mixture from sticking). Gently knead the dough for 5 to 10 minutes.

6. Form the dough into one large ball and place it in the center of the baking sheet. Press down on the ball with a lightly floured rolling pin, and create a flattened circle about 1½ inches thick.

7. Spread the chunky cranberry sauce evenly over the dough with a spoon, and sprinkle with chopped pecans.

8. Bake for 13 to 15 minutes, or until golden brown (inserted toothpick should come out clean). Slice into 6 pieces.

NUTRIENT ANALYSIS

♦ 1 SERVING = 1 SCONE

Calories: 219	Protein: 6.6 g	Carbohydrates: 38 g	Sugar: 2.3 g	Total fat: 4.3 g
Saturated fat: 0.7 g	Cholesterol: 2.4 mg	Sodium: 367 mg	Fiber: 2.3 g	Calcium: 147 mg

1,200-CALORIE PLAN

1 scone

1,400- & 1,600-CALORIE PLANS

1 scone
1 cup whole strawberries

1,800-CALORIE PLAN

1 scone
1 cup whole strawberries
¼ cup 1% low-fat cottage cheese or nonfat
   flavored yogurt

2,000-CALORIE PLAN

1 scone
1 cup whole strawberries
½ cup 1% low-fat cottage cheese or nonfat
   flavored yogurt

Low-Fat Granola

Serves 9

Most granolas are so high in oil that they have no place on a weight-management meal plan, but this one's satisfyingly crunchy and contains very little fat. The dried cranberries lend color, but if you can't find them, you can substitute raisins.

Vegetable cooking spray
1/4 cup dark brown sugar
1/4 cup water
2 teaspoons vanilla extract
1/2 teaspoon salt
4 cups old-fashioned rolled oats
1/2 cup dried cranberries
1/2 cup bran flakes
1/2 cup wheat flakes
1/4 cup Splenda

1. Preheat the oven to 275°. Spray a large baking sheet with cooking spray.

2. In a glass 2-cup measure, stir together the brown sugar and water. Microwave on high for 2 minutes. Stir again to dissolve the sugar. Stir in the vanilla and salt.

3. In a large mixing bowl, toss and thoroughly stir the oats with the sugar syrup. Spread the mixture on the baking sheet and bake for 30 to 40 minutes, stirring occasionally.

4. When the mixture is crunchy, remove from the oven. Stir in the dried cranberries, bran flakes, wheat flakes, and Splenda. Return to the oven for 8 to 10 more minutes, stirring once.

5. Remove the baking sheet from the oven. Allow the granola to cool completely on the baking sheet before storing in an airtight container.

◆ **1 SERVING = ¼ CUP**

Calories: 197	Protein: 5.3 g	Carbohydrates: 40 g	Sugar: 12 g	Total fat: 2.6 g
Saturated fat: 0 g	Cholesterol: 0 mg	Sodium: 164 mg	Fiber: 4.2 g	Calcium: 55 mg

1,200-CALORIE PLAN

1 serving granola, dry

1,400- & 1,600-CALORIE PLANS

1 serving granola
½ cup nonfat, flavored yogurt or ½ cup skim
  milk

1,800-CALORIE PLAN

1 serving granola
1 cup nonfat, flavored yogurt or 1 cup skim
  milk

2,000-CALORIE PLAN

1 serving granola
1 cup nonfat, flavored yogurt or 1 cup skim
  milk
1 peach or plum, or ½ grapefruit

Fruity Tofu Yogurt Shake

Serves 2

A meal in a glass that's meant for days when you want an energizing breakfast you can make in a flash. Be sure to use ripe, sweet strawberries and whirl the ingredients in a blender until the drink is pink and frothy.

4 ounces silken tofu
1 cup plain fat-free yogurt
1 cup sliced strawberries
1 tablespoon honey
1 tablespoon Splenda
½ teaspoon vanilla extract
¼ cup orange juice
3 ice cubes
2 whole strawberries, for garnish

1. In a blender, combine all the ingredients except the whole strawberries. Blend until smooth.

2. Pour into two tall glasses. Garnish each glass with a whole strawberry.

NUTRIENT ANALYSIS

◆ **1 SERVING = 1 SHAKE**

Calories: 198	Protein: 11 g	Carbohydrates: 34.7 g	Sugar: 27.7 g	Total fat: 2.4 g
Saturated fat: 0 g	Cholesterol: 2.2 mg	Sodium: 99 mg	Fiber: 3.7 g	Calcium: 302 mg

1,200-CALORIE PLAN

1 shake

1,400- & 1,600-CALORIE PLANS

1 shake
1 slice 40-calorie whole wheat bread, toasted

1,800-CALORIE PLAN

1 shake
2 slices 40-calorie whole bread, toasted
1 teaspoon peanut butter

2,000-CALORIE PLAN

1 shake
2 slices 40-calorie whole wheat bread,
  toasted
2 teaspoons peanut butter

Strawberry Yogurt Parfait

....

Serves 2

One of the easiest recipes in the chapter, this parfait is crunchy, creamy, and fruity all at the same time. Making it in a flute or parfait glass ensures that it's also beautiful to look at, since the layers of yogurt, strawberries, and granola offer a nice contrast of color and texture.

    8-ounces nonfat vanilla yogurt
    1 cup fresh strawberries, finely chopped
    ¼ cup low-fat granola
    2 whole strawberries, for garnish

1. Spoon 2 tablespoons of yogurt into a thin, clear flute or parfait glass.

2. Layer 1 to 2 tablespoons of strawberries on top of the yogurt. Then layer 1 to 2 tablespoons of granola on top of the strawberries. Repeat.

3. Top with a whole strawberry.

NUTRIENT ANALYSIS

♦ **1 SERVING = 1 PARFAIT**

Calories: 127	Protein: 6.5 g	Carbohydrates: 24 g	Sugar: 7.7 g	Total fat: 1.2 g
Saturated fat: 0 g	Cholesterol: 1.5 mg	Sodium: 96 mg	Fiber: 3 g	Calcium: 189 mg

1,200-CALORIE PLAN

1 parfait

1 egg, hard-boiled, poached, or scrambled
using cooking spray

1,400- & 1,600-CALORIE PLANS

1 parfait

1 egg, hard-boiled, poached, or scrambled
using cooking spray

1 slice 40-calorie whole wheat bread, toasted

1,800-CALORIE PLAN

1 parfait

1 egg, hard-boiled, poached, or scrambled
using cooking spray

1 slice 40-calorie whole wheat bread, toasted

1 slice fat-free cheese

2,000-CALORIE PLAN

1 parfait

1 egg, hard-boiled, poached, or scrambled
using cooking spray

2 slices 40-calorie whole wheat bread,
toasted

1 slice fat-free cheese

Five

Lunch: Our Midday Motivator

Southwestern Chicken Soup
Baba Ghanouj
Hummus
Red Lentil Dip with Crudités and Pita Wedges
Three-Cheese Quesadillas
Black Bean and Spinach Burritos
Egg White Vegetable Dijonnaise
Grilled Vegetable Sandwich
Boston Crab Salad Triangles
Cape Cod Tuna Salad
Cool Tabbouleh with Mint
Red Lentil and Bulgur Pilaf

By midday, our energy is flagging and we're starting to feel that hunger that occurs after a busy morning. It's time for a power lunch that will see you right through the afternoon and ensure that you don't feel sluggish halfway through. Whether you prefer lunch to be a hot-cooked meal, a quick sandwich, or a robust soup, this eclectic collection is sure to satisfy.

If you love soup, the Southwestern Chicken Soup is delicious, colorful, filling, and chock-full of healthful ingredients like red bell peppers, green split peas, chunks of boneless chicken breast, and a generous dose of salsa. Boston Crab Salad Triangles are just the thing to serve when you want something showy and elegant. And the dips—garlicky, lemony Baba Ghanouj, the nicely seasoned Red Lentil Dip with Crudités and Pita Wedges, and Hummus—make great picnic fare or the perfect meal to nibble on while you're sitting at a desk.

Whatever you choose, keep in mind that you should be eating roughly 300 calories for lunch if you are following the 1,200-calorie plan, about 350 calories if you are following the 1,400-calorie plan, approximately 400 calories for the 1,600-calorie plan, and 500 calories for both the 1,800- and 2,000-calorie plans. But don't feel overwhelmed with number crunching. Like all the meals, the math has been done for you. Find your appropriate portion breakdown underneath each recipe and enjoy your lunch!

Southwestern Chicken Soup

Serves 6

An abundance of spices goes into this anything-but-bland main course soup, which gets a lovely color from three different varieties of bell peppers, salsa, and yellow split peas. You may prepare both the soup and the tortilla strips a day ahead. Be sure to garnish the soup with the tortilla strips just before serving.

1½ teaspoons chili powder
¾ teaspoon ground coriander
¼ teaspoon salt
¼ teaspoon garlic powder
⅛ teaspoon ground chipotle chili pepper
⅛ teaspoon freshly ground black pepper
1 pound skinless, boneless chicken breast, cut into 4 pieces
Cooking spray
2 teaspoons olive oil
1 large onion, peeled and coarsely chopped
1 green bell pepper, peeled, seeded, and coarsely chopped
1 yellow bell pepper, peeled, seeded, and coarsely chopped
1 red bell pepper, peeled, seeded, and coarsely chopped
1 garlic clove, peeled and minced
2 cups fat-free chicken broth
2 cups water
½ cup yellow split peas
½ cup salsa
Juice of ½ lime
3 ten-inch flour tortillas
½ cup shredded, reduced-fat Monterey Jack cheese

1. In a small bowl, stir together the chili powder, coriander, salt, garlic powder, chili pepper, and black pepper. Coat all sides of the chicken pieces with the spice mixture.

2. Spray a large nonstick skillet with cooking spray. Add the olive oil and use a paper towel to distribute it evenly around the pan. Cook the chicken pieces over medium heat for 7 minutes then turn and cook for 6 minutes on the other side. Remove the chicken from the pan.

3. Add the onion, bell peppers, and garlic to the pan and sauté over medium heat for 5 minutes. Meanwhile, cut the chicken into thin strips.

4. Return the chicken to the pan, along with the broth, water, and split peas. Bring to a boil, reduce the heat, and simmer for ½ hour, partially covered; stir occasionally.

5. Add the salsa and lime juice and simmer for another 10 minutes. Remove from heat.

6. Preheat the oven to 400°. Cut the tortillas into thin strips (a pizza cutter works very well for this job). Spray a large baking sheet with cooking spray. Arrange the tortilla strips on the baking sheet. Bake for about 10 minutes, stirring occasionally, until crisp and golden brown.

7. Divide the soup among 6 bowls. Top each serving with ½ cup tortilla strips and 2 teaspoons grated Monterey Jack cheese.

NUTRIENT ANALYSIS

◆ **1 SERVING = 1⅓ CUPS SOUP + ½ CUP TORTILLA STRIPS AND 2 TEASPOONS CHEESE**

Calories: 248	Protein: 26 g	Carbohydrates: 19 g	Sugar: 1.7 g	Total fat: 8 g
Saturated fat: 3.4 g	Cholesterol: 57 mg	Sodium: 462 mg	Fiber: 2.4 g	Calcium: 188 mg

1,200-CALORIE PLAN

1 serving soup
1 cup baby carrots

1,600-CALORIE PLAN

1½ servings soup
Handful baby carrots (about 8)

1,400-CALORIE PLAN

1 serving soup
1 cup baby carrots
2 tablespoons low-fat salad dressing

1,800- & 2,000-CALORIE PLANS

2 servings soup
Handful baby carrots (about 8)

Baba Ghanouj

Serves 2

This Middle Eastern eggplant puree, nicely seasoned with garlic and lemon, can be used as a spread or a dip. You can prepare it a day ahead of time, but don't try to freeze leftovers.

2 large eggplants
2 cloves garlic, finely chopped
2 teaspoons tahini
Juice of 1 large lemon
2 teaspoons extra-virgin olive oil
2 teaspoons chopped onion
2 teaspoons oregano
Salt and freshly ground black pepper

1. Preheat the oven to 375°.

2. Pierce the eggplants with fork. Bake until soft and tender, about 30 to 40 minutes. Test with a toothpick.

3. Let the eggplants cool. Scoop the insides into bowl. Discard the skin. Mash the eggplant with a fork.

4. Add the remaining ingredients and mix.

5. Add salt and pepper to taste.

NUTRIENT ANALYSIS

♦ **1 SERVING = A BIT MORE THAN ¾ CUP**

Calories: 228	Protein: 6.9 g	Carbohydrates: 38.5 g	Sugar: 19 g	Total fat: 8.3 g
Saturated fat: 1.2 g	Cholesterol: 0 g	Sodium: 19 mg	Fiber: 14.75 g	Calcium: 76.8 mg

1,200-CALORIE PLAN

1 serving baba ghanouj

1 small whole wheat pita (no more than 70 calories), toasted

1,400-CALORIE PLAN

1 serving baba ghanouj

1 small whole wheat pita (no more than 70 calories), toasted

8 baby carrots and tomato slices

1,600-CALORIE PLAN

1 serving baba ghanouj

1 standard-size whole wheat pita (no more than 150 calories), toasted

1 cup raw carrots, celery, bell peppers, and cucumbers

1,800- & 2,000-CALORIE PLAN

1 cup baba ghanouj

1 standard-size whole wheat pita (no more than 150 calories), toasted

1 cup raw carrots, celery, bell peppers, and cucumbers

Hummus

. . . .

Serves 5

Lemon and garlic enliven this Middle Eastern classic dip, which is effortless to prepare in the food processor. Use the freshest garlic you can find, and prepare a day ahead if you like.

2 fifteen-ounce cans chickpeas (garbanzo beans), drained
½ cup tahini (sesame paste)
¼ cup lemon juice
2 cloves garlic
Salt and freshly ground black pepper

1. Place the chickpeas, tahini, lemon juice, and garlic in food processor. Blend until smooth.

2. Add small amounts of water (while blending) if the mixture is too thick.

3. Season with salt and pepper to taste

NUTRIENT ANALYSIS

◆ **1 SERVING = ½ CUP**

Calories: 279	Protein: 9.8 g	Carbohydrates: 31 g	Sugar: 0 g	Total fat: 14 g
Saturated fat: 1.9 g	Cholesterol: 0 mg	Sodium: 347 mg	Fiber: 6.14 g	Calcium: 72 mg

1,200-CALORIE PLAN

1 serving hummus
1 cup raw celery, cucumbers, bell peppers, zucchini, and broccoli

1,400-CALORIE PLAN

1 serving hummus
1 cup raw celery, cucumbers, bell peppers, zucchini, and broccoli
1 slice reduced-calorie whole wheat bread, toasted

1,600-CALORIE PLAN

1 serving hummus
1 cup raw carrots, celery, cucumbers, bell peppers, zucchini, and broccoli
1 small whole wheat pita, cut into triangles and toasted (any brand that's 70 calories or fewer)

1,800- & 2,000-CALORIE PLANS

1 serving hummus
2 cups raw carrots, celery, cucumbers, bell peppers, zucchini, and broccoli
1 standard whole wheat pita, cut into triangles and toasted (any brand that's 150 calories or fewer)

Red Lentil Dip with Crudités and Pita Wedges

Serves 10

Perfectly seasoned with exotic spices and mellowed with walnuts and olive oil, this delicious dip goes well both with toasted pita wedges and with crunchy raw vegetables. This keeps for a couple of days in the fridge.

DIP
1 cup dried small red lentils
2 bay leaves
1 tablespoon olive oil
1 medium onion, peeled and chopped
2 tablespoons walnuts
1½ tablespoons tomato paste
1½ teaspoons sea salt
¾ teaspoon ground cumin
1 teaspoon ground coriander
½ teaspoon ground caraway seeds
Pinch of ground red pepper
4 garlic cloves, peeled and minced
3 tablespoons lemon juice

PITA WEDGES
4 six-inch pitas, each cut into 6 wedges
Cooking spray
¼ teaspoon sea salt
20 baby carrots

1. Preheat the oven to 350°.

2. In a large saucepan, place the lentils and bay leaves with water to cover. Bring to a boil. Cover, reduce heat, and simmer for 10 minutes, or until the lentils are tender. Drain and discard the bay leaves.

3. In a medium nonstick skillet, heat the oil over medium heat. Add the onion and walnuts and stir-fry for 5 minutes. Add the tomato paste, sea salt, cumin, coriander, caraway seeds, red pepper, and garlic. Cook for 5 minutes. Stir in the lemon juice.

4. In food processor, combine the cooked lentils and the onion mixture. Process until smooth.

5. Sprinkle the pita wedges with sea salt. Arrange them in a single layer on a baking sheet sprayed with cooking spray. Bake for 15 minutes until golden.

6. Serve the dip with pita and baby carrots.

NUTRIENT ANALYSIS

◆ 1 SERVING = 3 TABLESPOONS DIP AND 2 PITA WEDGES

Calories: 171	Protein: 8 g	Carbohydrates: 28.5 g	Sugar: 4.3 g	Total fat: 3 g
Saturated fat: 0 g	Cholesterol: 0 mg	Sodium: 552 mg	Fiber: 7.4 g	Calcium: 46 mg

1,200-CALORIE PLAN

1 serving dip with 2 pita wedges
Unlimited crudités
1 peach, 1 plum, or 1 cup strawberries

1,400-CALORIE PLAN

1 serving dip with 4 pita wedges
Unlimited crudités
1 peach, 1 plum, or 1 cup strawberries

1,600-CALORIE PLAN

2 servings dip with 4 pita wedges
Unlimited crudités

1,800- & 2,000-CALORIE PLANS

2 servings dip with 6 pita wedges
Unlimited crudités
1 cup cubed pineapple, 1 apple, or 20 grapes

Three-Cheese Quesadillas

Serves 2

This savory quesadilla made healthy by using fat-free cheese has crunch and color thanks to the fresh veggies. When shopping for tortillas, make sure to choose the six-inch ones, not the much larger size that have too many calories.

Cooking oil spray
2 six-inch low-fat flour tortillas (bonus if you buy whole wheat)
1 garlic clove, peeled and finely minced
1 teaspoon chopped fresh Italian parsley
2 tablespoons chopped tomato
2 tablespoons chopped yellow bell pepper
2 ounces grated fat-free cheddar cheese
2 ounces grated fat-free mozzarella cheese
2 tablespoons freshly grated Parmesan cheese

1. Lightly spray an 8- or 10-inch nonstick skillet with cooking spray. Cook each tortilla over medium heat, turning once, for 1 minute per side. Transfer the tortillas to a plate.

2. Sprinkle half of each tortilla with garlic and parsley. Top with the tomato, bell pepper, cheddar, mozzarella, and Parmesan. Fold the tortillas in half to cover the filling.

3. Spray the skillet with more cooking spray. Turn the heat to medium. Place the quesadillas in the skillet and cook them for 2 to 3 minutes per side, turning once, until the cheese is melted. Cut each quesadilla in half.

NUTRIENT ANALYSIS

◆ **1 SERVING = 1 QUESADILLA**

Calories: 274	Protein: 21 g	Carbohydrates: 39.5 g	Sugar: 0.4 g	Total fat: 4.1 g
Saturated fat: 1.5 g	Cholesterol: 2 mg	Sodium: 911 mg	Fiber: 2.65 g	Calcium: 376 mg

1,200-CALORIE PLAN

1 quesadilla

1 cup raw celery, peppers, cucumbers, and cherry tomatoes

1,400-CALORIE PLAN

1 quesadilla

Mixed vegetable salad with unlimited lettuce, tomatoes, carrots, onions, peppers, mushrooms, celery, and cucumbers

2 tablespoons low-fat or fat-free salad dressing

1,600-CALORIE PLAN

1 quesadilla

Mixed vegetable salad with unlimited lettuce, tomatoes, carrots, onions, peppers, mushrooms, celery, and cucumbers, and 1 rounded tablespoon beans (chickpeas, black beans, kidney, etc.)

2 tablespoons low-fat or fat-free salad dressing

1,800- & 2,000-CALORIE PLANS

1½ quesadillas

Mixed vegetable salad with unlimited lettuce, tomatoes, carrots, onions, peppers, mushrooms, celery, and cucumbers

2 tablespoons low-fat or fat-free salad dressing

Black Bean and Spinach Burritos

Serves 2

Instead of high-fat ground beef, these Southwestern-flavored tortillas are filled with seasoned black beans and spinach. But they're not just for vegetarians—you'll be pleasantly surprised at how satisfying they are. You can wilt the spinach in the microwave instead of on top of the stove. (You may use leftover black beans in place of the cannellini beans in the Vegetable and White Bean Salad in the next chapter.)

4 cups fresh spinach, leaves only, washed and stemmed
Vegetable oil cooking spray
1/2 fifteen-ounce can black beans, rinsed and drained
1/4 cup salsa
Pinch of ground cumin
Pinch of chili powder
2 six-inch low-fat flour tortillas
4 tablespoons nonfat sour cream
1 teaspoon freshly squeezed lime juice
1/2 cup grated nonfat Monterey Jack cheese
1 plum tomato, chopped
1 scallion, thinly sliced

1. Bring a large pot of water to the boil. Add the spinach and cook for 1 minute. Remove and drain well in a colander, pressing out as much liquid as possible.

2. Preheat the oven to 350°. Spray a shallow baking dish with cooking spray.

3. In small bowl, stir together the spinach, black beans, salsa, cumin, and chili powder. Divide the mixture between the two tortillas, spreading it down the middle of each. Roll the tortillas around the filling. Place the tortillas, seam side down, in the baking dish. Bake for 15 minutes.

4. In a small bowl, stir together the sour cream and lime juice. Spread this evenly over the burritos. Top with the grated Monterey Jack, chopped tomatoes, and sliced scallions. Bake an additional 5 minutes.

◆ **1 SERVING = 1 BURRITO**

Calories: 380	Protein: 27 g	Carbohydrates: 57 g	Sugar: 3.9 g	Total fat: 3.8 g

Saturated fat: 0.5 g	Cholesterol: 2.5 mg	Sodium: 1237 mg	Fiber: 14.6 g	Calcium: 517 mg

1,200-CALORIE PLAN

1 burrito (without cheese or sour cream)

1,400-CALORIE PLAN

1 burrito (without sour cream)

1,600-CALORIE PLAN

1 burrito
1 cup raw carrots, cucumbers, celery, and bell peppers

1,800- & 2,000-CALORIE PLANS

1 burrito
Mixed vegetable salad with unlimited lettuce, tomatoes, carrots, onions, peppers, mushrooms, celery, and cucumbers
2 tablespoons low-fat or fat-free salad dressing
$1/2$ grapefruit, 1 plum, or 1 tangerine

Egg White Vegetable Dijonnaise

Serves 2

This chunky egg salad gets both color and flavor from Dijon mustard and chopped fresh tomato. It makes a light, cooling meal on a warm day. If you want to get a head start, hard-boil the eggs ahead of time and chill them, and wash and refrigerate the salad greens, too. You may also want to try adding a little chopped dill.

8 eggs
2 tablespoons minced onion
½ tomato, finely chopped
1 tablespoon low-fat mayonnaise
2 tablespoons Dijon mustard
2 tablespoons Mrs. Dash low-sodium seasoning
Salt and freshly ground black pepper

1. Boil the eggs in salted water for 10 + minutes.

2. Immediately run the boiled eggs under cool water, crack, and peel away shells. The eggs will peel easier if you leave them under the running water.

3. Separate the whites from the yolks and discard the yolks.

4. In a large mixing bowl, chop the egg whites to desired consistency. Add the onion, tomato, mayonnaise, mustard, Mrs. Dash, and salt and pepper to taste.

5. Serve on a large bed of greens.

NUTRIENT ANALYSIS

◆ **1 SERVING = ½ PORTION (4 EGG WHITES)**

Calories: 96	Protein: 14.7 g	Carbohydrates: 12 g	Sugar: 2.6 g	Total fat: 1 g
Saturated fat: 0 g	Cholesterol: 0 mg	Sodium: 320 mg	Fiber: 0.6 g	Calcium: 18 mg

1,200-CALORIE PLAN

1 serving egg salad

1 whole wheat English muffin, toasted

Mixed vegetable salad with unlimited lettuce, tomatoes, carrots, onions, peppers, mushrooms, celery, and cucumbers

2 tablespoons low-fat or fat-free salad dressing

1,400-CALORIE PLAN

$1^1/_2$ servings egg salad

1 whole wheat English muffin, toasted

Mixed vegetable salad with unlimited lettuce, tomatoes, carrots, onions, peppers, mushrooms, celery, and cucumbers

2 tablespoons low-fat or fat-free salad dressing

1,600-CALORIE PLAN

$1^1/_2$ servings egg salad

1 whole wheat English muffin, toasted

Mixed vegetable salad with unlimited lettuce, tomatoes, carrots, onions, peppers, mushrooms, celery, and cucumbers

2 tablespoons low-fat or fat-free salad dressing

$1/_2$ grapefruit or 1 plum

1,800- & 2,000-CALORIE PLANS

2 servings (whole portion) egg salad

1 whole wheat English muffin, toasted

Mixed vegetable salad with unlimited lettuce, tomatoes, carrots, onions, peppers, mushrooms, celery, and cucumbers

2 tablespoons low-fat or fat-free salad dressing

1 small banana, 1 apple, or $1/_2$ cantaloupe

Grilled Vegetable Sandwich

Serves 2

This sandwich always wins rave reviews for its colorful appearance, meaty, satisfying taste, and wonderful flavor imparted by the fresh basil. You can make the dressing ahead of time and store it in a covered container in the refrigerator.

1 tablespoon Dijon mustard
1 teaspoon deli mustard
⅓ cup nonfat plain yogurt
Freshly ground black pepper
1 tablespoon minced onion
¼ teaspoon garlic powder
½ teaspoon fresh lemon juice
1 tablespoon nonfat cottage cheese
½ small summer squash, thinly sliced
½ small eggplant, thinly sliced
½ small zucchini, thinly sliced
½ small red onion, thinly sliced
1 teaspoon dried oregano
Pinch of cayenne pepper
Vegetable oil cooking spray
2 standard hamburger buns (preferably whole wheat)
2 slices roasted red pepper from a jar
½ tomato, sliced
6 fresh basil leaves

1. Preheat the oven broiler.

2. Prepare the dressing: In a blender, combine both mustards, yogurt, pepper, onion, garlic powder, lemon juice, and cottage cheese. Process until smooth.

3. Arrange the squash, eggplant, zucchini, and red onion in a single layer on a baking sheet. Sprinkle with the oregano and cayenne pepper. Spray with cooking spray. Broil the vegetables

for 5 to 7 minutes, until golden brown. Turn the vegetables over and broil on the other side for 5 minutes. Remove from the oven.

4. Split the hamburger buns in half and toast them for 30 to 40 seconds under the broiler.

5. On the bottom halves, place a slice of roasted red pepper, half the tomato slices, and 3 basil leaves. Arrange the slices of grilled vegetables over this. Spread the dressing on the top halves. Place these on top of the vegetables. Cut each sandwich in half.

NUTRIENT ANALYSIS

♦ **1 SERVING = ½ VEGETABLES WITH FULL HAMBURGER BUN**

| Calories: 191 | Protein: 9.2 g | Carbohydrates: 36 g | Sugar: 11 g | Total fat: 2.8 g |

| Saturated fat: 0 g | Cholesterol: 0 mg | Sodium: 314 mg | Fiber: 8 g | Calcium: 166 mg |

1,200-CALORIE PLAN

1 sandwich
8-ounce container nonfat, flavored yogurt (any brand 120 calories or fewer)

1,400-CALORIE PLAN

1 sandwich
8-ounce container of nonfat, flavored yogurt (any brand 120 calories or fewer)
½ grapefruit, 1 clementine, or 1 cup whole strawberries

1,600-CALORIE PLAN

1 sandwich
8-ounce container of nonfat, flavored yogurt (any brand 120 calories or fewer)
½ cantaloupe, 1 apple, or 1 cup blueberries

1,800- & 2,000-CALORIE PLANS

1 sandwich
8-ounce container of nonfat, flavored yogurt (any brand 120 calories or fewer)
2 tablespoons slivered almonds, or 3 tablespoons wheat germ or low-fat granola
½ cantaloupe, 1 apple, or 1 cup blueberries

Boston Crab Salad Triangles

Serves 4 (4 triangles each)

This salad is quick, elegant, and pretty—perfect for a ladies' lunch. Stuffing it into a whole wheat pita bumps up the fiber content, and lettuce and tomato add volume, crunch, and color.

16 ounces Alaska king crab (or imitation flaked crab)
4 tablespoons low-fat mayonnaise
1 tablespoon Mrs. Dash low-sodium seasoning
2 teaspoons minced onion
4 standard whole wheat pitas
Lettuce and tomato (optional)

1. In a food processor, shred the crab.

2. In a large bowl, thoroughly mix the shredded crab with low-fat mayo, Mrs. Dash, and minced onion.

3. Slice each pita into four triangles and place in the oven until lightly toasted.

4. Gently layer lettuce and thinly sliced tomato inside each triangle pocket. Spoon the crab salad on top of pita triangles. (You may also prefer to stuff the crab salad inside with lettuce and tomato.)

NUTRIENT ANALYSIS

◆ **1 SERVING = ¾ CUP CRAB SALAD AND 4 PITA TRIANGLES**

Calories: 314	Protein: 20 g	Carbohydrates: 56 g	Sugar: 6 g	Total fat: 4 g
Saturated fat: 0.5 g	Cholesterol: 23 mg	Sodium: 1436 mg	Fiber: 5 g	Calcium: 28 mg

1,200-CALORIE PLAN

1 serving crab salad
4 pita triangles

1,400-CALORIE PLAN

1⅓ servings (1 cup) crab salad
4 pita triangles

1,600-CALORIE PLAN

1⅓ servings (1 cup) crab salad
4 pita triangles
16 baby carrots (2 handfuls)

1,800- & 2,000-CALORIE PLANS

1⅓ servings (1 cup) crab salad
4 pita triangles
16 baby carrots
1 sliced apple or 1 cup cubed pineapple

Cape Cod Tuna Salad

Serves 1

This creative tuna salad gets its tangy flavor and pretty color from the dried cranberries and chopped apple. Serve it over your favorite greens for a lunch that won't leave you feeling hungry an hour later.

1 can (6 ounces) water-packed tuna
1 tablespoon low-fat mayonnaise
2 teaspoons dried cranberries (cran-raisins)
½ scallion, chopped
¼ fuji apple, peeled and finely chopped
Salt and freshly ground black pepper

Drain the tuna and mash it with a fork. Mix in all ingredients, and serve over a bed of greens (no extra dressing).

NUTRIENT ANALYSIS

Calories: 281	Protein: 40 g	Carbohydrates: 14 g	Sugar: 11.7 g	Total fat: 6.1 g
Saturated fat: 1.4 g	Cholesterol: 71 mg	Sodium: 782 mg	Fiber: 1.4 g	Calcium: 31 mg

1,200-CALORIE PLAN

1 serving tuna salad

Bed of greens with onion and cucumber

1,400-CALORIE PLAN

1 serving tuna salad

Bed of greens with onion and cucumber

1 slice 40-calorie whole wheat bread, toasted

1,600-CALORIE PLAN

1 serving tuna salad

Bed of greens with onion and cucumber

1 slice 40-calorie whole wheat bread, toasted

$1\frac{1}{2}$ cups whole strawberries or 1 orange

1,800- & 2,000-CALORIE PLANS

1 serving tuna salad

Bed of greens with onion, tomato, and
cucumber

2 slices 40-calorie whole wheat bread,
toasted

1 apple or $\frac{3}{4}$ cup blueberries

Cool Tabbouleh with Mint

Serves 4

This refreshing salad is redolent of garden vegetables: fresh mint, parsley, chopped tomatoes, and red onion. For the best flavor, be sure to remove from the refrigerator a half hour or so before serving.

1 cup bulgur
2 cups minced fresh parsley (stems removed)
1 cup minced fresh mint leaves
2 medium tomatoes, peeled, seeded, and chopped
1 small red onion, peeled and chopped
¼ cup olive oil
5 tablespoons freshly squeezed lemon juice
Salt and freshly ground black pepper
2 cups romaine lettuce leaves, washed and crisped

1. Cover the bulgur in water and soak for 15 to 20 minutes. Drain and squeeze well to get out as much water as possible.

2. In a large serving bowl, combine the bulgur with the parsley, mint, tomatoes, red onion, and olive oil. Sprinkle on the lemon juice. Season to taste with salt and pepper. Refrigerate until shortly before serving time. Arrange the tabbouleh on lettuce leaves and serve at room temperature.

NUTRIENT ANALYSIS

◆ 1 SERVING = ¼ OF THE RECIPE

Calories: 288	Protein: 7 g	Carbohydrates: 37 g	Sugar: 4.7 g	Total fat: 14.5 g
Saturated fat: 1.9 g	Cholesterol: 0 g	Sodium: 615 mg	Fiber: 10 g	Calcium: 91 mg

1,200-CALORIE PLAN

1 serving tabbouleh

Sliced cucumber

1,400-CALORIE PLAN

1 serving tabbouleh

Sliced cucumber

$1/2$ cup blueberries or 1 peach

1,600-CALORIE PLAN

1 serving tabbouleh

Sliced cucumber and 1 cup baby carrots

$1/2$ cup blueberries or 1 peach

1,800- & 2,000-CALORIE PLANS

$1^1/2$ servings tabbouleh

Sliced cucumber

$1/2$ cup blueberries or 1 peach

Red Lentil and Bulgur Pilaf

Serves 6

This thick, restorative, and filling dish is a good choice when you want to eat something vegetarian. Be sure to use dried mint as specified in the recipe, as the flavor is more intense than that of fresh. The chopped fresh mint works nicely as a garnish.

1 tablespoon olive oil
1 large Spanish onion, peeled and finely diced
3 garlic cloves, peeled and minced
2 tablespoons tomato paste
1 medium tomato, peeled, seeded, and chopped
1 tablespoon paprika
Pinch of ground red pepper
1½ cups red lentils
¼ cup long-grain white rice
2 cups chicken broth
4½ cups water
¼ cup bulgur
1 tablespoon dried mint
1 teaspoon salt, or to taste
¼ teaspoon freshly ground black pepper
½ cup packaged croutons
1½ teaspoons fresh mint, for garnish
6 lemon wedges, for garnish

1. In a heavy medium saucepan, heat the olive oil over medium heat. Add the onion and garlic and cook for 2 or 3 minutes. When the onions are soft, add the tomato paste, chopped tomato, paprika, ground red pepper, lentils, rice, broth, and water.

2. Cover the pan and bring to a boil. Lower the heat and simmer for 25 to 30 minutes, stirring occasionally, until the rice is tender.

3. Add the bulgur, mint, salt, and pepper. Cook for 10 minutes, stirring occasionally.

4. Serve topped with chopped fresh mint. Garnish with lemon wedges.

◆ **1 SERVING = ⅙ OF RECIPE**

| Calories: 285 | Protein: 19 g | Carbohydrates: 48.6 g | Sugar: 5.2 g | Total fat: 4 g |
| Saturated fat: 0 g | Cholesterol: 8.3 mg | Sodium: 521 mg | Fiber: 18.7 g | Calcium: 77 mg |

1,200-CALORIE PLAN

1 serving pilaf
1 large portobello mushroom, marinated in
   balsamic vinegar and broiled

1,400-CALORIE PLAN

1 serving pilaf
Mixed vegetable salad with unlimited lettuce,
   tomatoes, carrots, onions, peppers,
   mushrooms, celery, and cucumbers
2 tablespoons low-fat or fat-free salad
   dressing

1,600-CALORIE PLAN

1 serving pilaf
Mixed vegetable salad with unlimited lettuce,
   tomatoes, carrots, onions, peppers,
   mushrooms, celery, and cucumbers
2 tablespoons low-fat or fat-free salad
   dressing
½ grapefruit, 1 orange, 1 plum, or 1 peach

1,800- & 2,000-CALORIE PLANS

1½ servings pilaf
Mixed vegetable salad with unlimited lettuce,
   tomatoes, carrots, onions, peppers,
   mushrooms, celery, and cucumbers
2 tablespoons low-fat or fat-free salad
   dressing

Six

Dinner Is Served

Chicken and Cashew Lettuce Wraps
Chicken Dijon
Chicken Mushroom Marinara
Crunchy Chicken Strips with Honey Mustard Dipping Sauce
Honey Ginger Chicken Stir-Fry
Veronica's Chicken Paprika
Extra-Lean Turkey Chili
Microwave Stuffed Peppers
Portobello Turkey Loaf
Shepherd's Pie with Cauliflower and Turkey
Southwestern Turkey Meat Loaf
Tex-Mex Turkey Burgers
Turkey Loaf with the Kitchen Sink
Herb-Marinated Flank Steak
Slow-Cooker Beef Stroganoff
Pork Lo Mein
Asian Citrus Salmon Steak
Honey Mustard Salmon
Maple-Glazed Salmon
Lemon Pepper–Seared Tuna Steaks
Shrimp with Garlic and Feta
Spicy Jambalaya
Angel Hair Pasta Piccata
Cold Sesame Noodles

Baked Cauliflower Puree
Spinach-Cheese Timbale
Vegetable and White Bean Salad
Black Bean Soup with Sherry and Garlic

It's the meal we all look forward to at the end of a long day, when we want to relax, kick back, and enjoy a leisurely time with family and friends. With this varied, nutrient-packed, and exciting collection of recipes, you'll be able to create meals for everyone to enjoy as opposed to cooking one thing for them and something else for yourself (in which case you're sorely tempted to taste theirs anyway!).

Your portion size depends on which 90/10 plan you are following, but of course your friends and family can enjoy unlimited portions of these easy-to-make, delicious dishes. If you're cooking for yourself, wrap and freeze individual servings of appropriate recipes for future meals.

As usual, following each recipe are the absolute specific breakdowns for your personal plan. If you are on the 1,200-calorie plan, prepare to eat 350 calories for dinner. Those on the 1,400-calorie plan may eat 450 calories. For those on the 1,600- and 1,800-calorie plans, the allowance for dinner is 550 calories, and for those on the 2,000-calorie plan, the dinner allowance is 650 calories.

Here in this chapter, you'll find succulent beef dishes like the Herb-Marinated Flank Steak, chicken dishes to suit every taste, from a rich Chicken Dijon to a more casual Crunchy Chicken Strips with Honey Mustard Dipping Sauce. And if you're a vegetarian, you'll love Black Bean Soup with Sherry and Garlic and Cold Sesame Noodles.

Some of these dishes (like Angel Hair Pasta Piccata) are ready in minutes, and most recipes can be put together in under an hour. The one feature all these dishes have in common is that they are nutritious and satisfying. And if you need something further just because you feel like munching, remember that you can always have some extra crunchy raw or plain, cooked vegetables.

Chicken and Cashew Lettuce Wraps

Serves 6

Fun finger food for kids and grown-ups, this Asian-style "wrap" is made by scooping up the chicken mixture with crisp lettuce leaves. The cashews and water chestnuts give it some extra crunch.

1½ pounds boneless, chicken breast tenderloins
16 ounces canned water chestnuts
1 cup fat-free chicken broth
4 tablespoons low-sodium soy sauce
1 teaspoon cornstarch
2 tablespoons sesame oil
1 teaspoon ground ginger
1 tablespoon chopped garlic
1 egg white
3 tablespoons low-sodium teriyaki sauce
4 tablespoons unsalted whole cashews
1 head iceberg lettuce, chilled

1. Dice the chicken into small pieces and set aside in a large bowl. Chop up the water chestnuts and mix with the chicken pieces.

2. In a separate bowl, thoroughly mix the chicken broth, soy sauce, cornstarch, 1 tablespoon sesame oil, ginger, garlic, and egg white. Pour over the chicken and chestnuts. Cover and let marinate for 30 + minutes in the refrigerator.

3. Pour the chicken mixture into a large saucepan and cook over a medium-high flame, stirring continuously, until the liquid is absorbed and the chicken is cooked through.

4. Add the teriyaki sauce, remaining sesame oil, and cashews. Continue mixing over heat.

5. Scoop the chicken onto chilled whole lettuce leaves and roll up like a wrap.

♦ **1 SERVING = ¾ CUP CHICKEN MIXTURE + UNLIMITED LETTUCE LEAVES**

Calories: 286	Protein: 25.4 g	Carbohydrates: 17.4 g	Sugar: 4.6 g	Total fat: 16 g

Saturated fat: 3.5 g	Cholesterol: 94 mg	Sodium: 669 mg	Fiber: 1.4 g	Calcium: 21 mg

1,200-CALORIE PLAN

1 serving chicken
1 cup cubed pineapple or 1 cup fresh berries

1,400-CALORIE PLAN

1 serving chicken
½ cup cooked brown rice
1 orange or ½ grapefruit

1,600- & 1,800-CALORIE PLANS

1 serving chicken
1 cup cooked brown rice
1 orange or ½ grapefruit

2,000-CALORIE PLAN

1 serving chicken
1½ cups cooked brown rice
1 orange or ½ grapefruit

Chicken Dijon

Serves 6

A creamy sauce lightly flavored with Dijon mustard binds tender boneless chicken and steamed broccoli florets. This is a family-pleasing dish that can be made several hours ahead of time and reheated over low heat.

Cooking spray
6 five-ounce chicken breasts, cut into pieces
2 cups broccoli florets (fresh or frozen)
1 can low-fat cream of mushroom soup
1 cup skim milk
2 tablespoons Dijon mustard
½ cup grated low-fat sharp cheddar cheese

1. Coat a large frying pan with cooking spray. Sauté the chicken pieces until they are thoroughly cooked and lightly browned on both sides.

2. Microwave or steam the broccoli. Drain and add to the chicken.

3. In a bowl, thoroughly mix the mushroom soup, skim milk, mustard, and cheese; otherwise, soup will be clumpy.

4. Add the soup mixture to the chicken, bring to a boil, and simmer for 5 to 10 minutes.

NUTRIENT ANALYSIS

◆ **1 SERVING = 1 CUP**

Calories: 271	Protein: 41 g	Carbohydrates: 17.5 g	Sugar: 3.8 g	Total fat: 6.4 g
Saturated fat: 2.8 g	Cholesterol: 93 mg	Sodium: 816 mg	Fiber: 2 g	Calcium: 245 mg

1,200-CALORIE PLAN

1 serving chicken
$\frac{1}{2}$ cup cooked brown rice

1,400-CALORIE PLAN

1 serving chicken
$\frac{3}{4}$ cup cooked brown rice

1,600- & 1,800-CALORIE PLANS

1$\frac{1}{2}$ servings chicken
$\frac{3}{4}$ cup cooked brown rice

2,000-CALORIE PLAN

1$\frac{1}{2}$ servings chicken
1 cup cooked brown rice

Chicken Mushroom Marinara

Serves 6

This may be the easiest recipe you've ever made. Two kinds of mushrooms give this robust chicken marinara an exotic flavor. There's no need to sauté the meat first. Just add it to the hot sauce and let it simmer until done.

1½ jars (39 ounces) marinara sauce (any brand 50 calories or fewer per ½-cup serving)
1½ pounds chicken breast tenderloins, cut in half
4 large portobello mushrooms, sliced in thick strips
2 cups small white mushrooms, whole

1. In a saucepan, heat the marinara sauce over a low flame. Add the chicken and the mushrooms.

2. Bring the mixture to a boil. Cover and cook over medium heat for 1 hour, stirring every 10 minutes.

NUTRIENT ANALYSIS

♦ **1 SERVING = ⅙ OF THE RECIPE**

Calories: 259	Protein: 25.6 g	Carbohydrates: 17.5 g	Sugar: 6 g	Total fat: 0.9 g
Saturated fat: 2.5 g	Cholesterol: 94 mg	Sodium: 793 mg	Fiber: 6.8 g	Calcium: 56 mg

1,200-CALORIE PLAN

1 serving chicken

$^1/_2$ cup cooked whole wheat pasta

1,400-CALORIE PLAN

1 serving chicken

1 cup cooked whole wheat pasta

1,600- & 1,800-CALORIE PLANS

1 serving chicken

$1^1/_2$ cups cooked whole wheat pasta

2,000-CALORIE PLAN

$1^1/_2$ servings chicken

$1^1/_4$ cups cooked whole wheat pasta

Crunchy Chicken Strips with Honey Mustard Dipping Sauce

Serves 5

A tangy, easy-to-make sauce is perfect to serve with these cornmeal-dipped chicken fingers. Make the honey mustard sauce a day ahead, keep refrigerated, and use in place of high-fat butter next time you make a sandwich.

HONEY MUSTARD DIPPING SAUCE
¼ cup fat-free sour cream
¼ cup fat-free plain yogurt
2 tablespoons Dijon mustard
2 teaspoons honey

CHICKEN
1¼ pounds boneless, skinless chicken breast
⅔ cup cornmeal
¾ teaspoon salt
¾ teaspoon chili powder
1 egg
1 tablespoon water
Cooking spray
1 tablespoon olive oil

1. Make the honey mustard dipping sauce: In a small bowl, stir together the sour cream, yogurt, mustard, and honey. Cover and refrigerate.

2. Trim any visible fat from the chicken breasts and cut into strips. Pound them lightly to flatten.

3. In a small bowl, stir together the cornmeal, salt, and chili powder. In a shallow bowl, lightly beat the egg. Add the water and beat again.

4. Dip chicken pieces into the egg mixture and then into the cornmeal mixture, coating well.

5. Spray a large nonstick skillet with cooking spray. Add the olive oil. Over medium heat, cook the chicken for several minutes per side, turning once, until thoroughly cooked and golden brown. Serve with honey-mustard dipping sauce.

NUTRIENT ANALYSIS

♦ **1 SERVING = 4–6 PIECES**

Calories: 306	Protein: 25 g	Carbohydrates: 21 g	Sugar: 3.7 g	Total fat: 13.6 g
Saturated fat: 3.2 g	Cholesterol: 137 mg	Sodium: 472 mg	Fiber: 1.4 g	Calcium: 64 mg

1,200-CALORIE PLAN

1 serving chicken and sauce

Mixed vegetable salad with lettuce, onions, peppers, mushrooms, celery, and cucumbers

2 tablespoons low-fat or fat-free salad dressing

1,400-CALORIE PLAN

1 serving chicken and sauce

Mixed vegetable salad with lettuce, onions, peppers, mushrooms, celery, and cucumbers, with $1/4$ cup beans (any type)

2 tablespoons low-fat or fat-free salad dressing

1,600- & 1,800-CALORIE PLANS

$1^1/2$ servings chicken and sauce

Mixed vegetable salad with lettuce, onions, peppers, mushrooms, celery, and cucumbers, with $1/4$ cup beans (any type)

2 tablespoons low-fat or fat-free salad dressing

2,000-CALORIE PLAN

2 servings chicken and sauce

Mixed vegetable salad with lettuce, onions, peppers, mushrooms, celery, and cucumbers

2 tablespoons low-fat or fat-free salad dressing.

Honey Ginger Chicken Stir-Fry

Serves 4

A sweet-sour marinade enlivens this satisfying stir-fry, which pairs crisp, fresh green beans with morsels of chicken. It's crucial to use fresh ginger, not the dried ginger in a jar.

½ cup honey
⅓ cup low-sodium soy sauce
¼ cup lime and lemon juice (mixed)
1 tablespoon orange juice
½ teaspoon ground fresh ginger
20 ounces chicken breasts, cut into pieces
2 cups fresh green beans, washed and trimmed

1. In a bowl, combine the honey, soy sauce, lime and lemon juice, orange juice, and ginger.

2. Thoroughly coat the chicken pieces with the mixture, and place in a ziplock bag or covered bowl. Allow the chicken to marinate for at least 30 minutes.

3. In a separate bowl, steam or microwave the green beans until they are slightly soft. Drain and set aside.

4. In a large frying pan, pour in chicken, green beans, and extra marinade. Cook on a medium-high flame, stirring continuously, until the chicken is thoroughly cooked, about 6 to 8 minutes.

NUTRIENT ANALYSIS

◆ **1 SERVING = ¼ OF RECIPE**

Calories: 324	Protein: 35 g	Carbohydrates: 43 g	Sugar: 38 g	Total fat: 1.9 g
Saturated fat: 0.5 g	Cholesterol: 82 mg	Sodium: 887 mg	Fiber: 2.35 g	Calcium: 52.6 mg

1,200-CALORIE PLAN

1 serving stir-fry

1 cup steamed red and yellow peppers

1,400-CALORIE PLAN

1 serving stir-fry

½ cup cooked brown rice or whole wheat
  pasta

1,600- & 1,800-CALORIE PLANS

1 serving stir-fry

1 cup cooked brown rice or whole wheat
  pasta

2,000-CALORIE PLAN

1½ servings stir-fry

¾ cup cooked brown rice or whole wheat
  pasta

Veronica's Chicken Paprika

Serves 2

A terrific cook named Veronica generously provided me with this Hungarian recipe. She's become very health-conscious and has modified her original dish so that it's nutritious as well as flavorful. Thank you, Veronica!

¾ pound skinless, boneless chicken breast, cut into small chunks
2 tablespoons reduced-fat, soft tub margarine
1 large white onion, finely chopped
½ teaspoon salt
2 heaping teaspoons paprika
14–16 ounces low-fat chicken broth
2 medium tomatoes
2 medium green peppers, cut in half with seeds removed
1–2 teaspoons cornstarch
Salt and freshly ground black pepper

1. Place the chicken chunks in cold water to soak. Cover and set aside.

2. In a large skillet, heat the margarine over a medium flame. Add the chopped onions and sauté until soft and glassy. Add the salt and paprika. Stir thoroughly.

3. Drain the water from the chicken. Add the chicken to the skillet. Turn the chicken several times in order to begin cooking all sides.

4. Add the chicken broth and continue to stir. Add the whole tomatoes, pepper halves, and cornstarch. Cook until the chicken is soft and thoroughly cooked (remove one piece and slice through to test). Add salt and pepper to taste.

5. Divide into 2 servings: Each plate should have 2 half peppers, 1 whole tomato, and half the chicken-onion mixture.

◆ **1 SERVING = 1½ CUPS**

Calories: 340	Protein: 43.4 g	Carbohydrates: 18 g	Sugar: 6.3 g	Total fat: 10 g

Saturated fat: 2 g	Cholesterol: 98 mg	Sodium: 1782 mg	Fiber: 3.1 g	Calcium: 40 mg

1,200-CALORIE PLAN

1 serving chicken
Sliced cucumber

1,400-CALORIE PLAN

1 serving chicken
Mixed vegetable salad with unlimited lettuce,
   tomatoes, carrots, onions, peppers,
   mushrooms, celery, and cucumbers
2 tablespoons low-fat or fat-free salad
   dressing
½ grapefruit

1,600- & 1,800-CALORIE PLANS

1 serving chicken
½ cup cooked brown rice
Mixed vegetable salad with unlimited lettuce,
   tomatoes, carrots, onions, peppers,
   mushrooms, celery, and cucumbers
2 tablespoons low-fat or fat-free salad
   dressing

2,000-CALORIE PLAN

1½ servings chicken
½ cup cooked brown rice
Sliced cucumber

Extra-Lean Turkey Chili

Serves 8

You won't miss the beef in this hearty, well-seasoned dish, which relies on extra-lean ground turkey and kidney beans for its thick, crowd-pleasing consistency. If you love spicy foods, just sprinkle in a little extra ground red pepper. This one is my husband's specialty—an Ian Bauer original!

2 pounds extra-lean ground turkey breast
12 ounces crushed tomatoes (without paste)
12 ounces water
2 teaspoons garlic powder
1 teaspoons paprika
1 teaspoon cumin
1 teaspoon oregano
6 teaspoons chili powder
1 teaspoon salt
1 teaspoon freshly ground black pepper
½ onion, diced
½ teaspoon ground red pepper (add more for hotter chili)
2 teaspoons flour
1 can (15 ounces) red kidney beans

1. Brown the ground turkey in a skillet. Drain the fat.

2. Add the tomatoes, water, garlic powder, paprika, cumin, oregano, chili powder, salt, pepper, and onion. Mix thoroughly.

3. Cover the skillet and simmer for 25 to 30 minutes, stirring every 10 minutes.

4. Stir in the flour. Add the kidney beans.

5. Simmer, uncovered, for 20 minutes.

◆ **1 SERVING = 1 CUP**

Calories: 230	Protein: 30 g	Carbohydrates: 14 g	Sugar: 2.9 g	Total fat: 6 g

Saturated fat 1 g	Cholesterol: 55 mg	Sodium: 741 mg	Fiber: 5.4 g	Calcium: 54 mg

1,200-CALORIE PLAN

1 serving chili

Mixed vegetable salad with unlimited lettuce, tomatoes, carrots, onions, peppers, mushrooms, celery, and cucumbers

2 tablespoons low-fat or fat-free salad dressing

1,400-CALORIE PLAN

1 serving chili

Mixed vegetable salad with unlimited lettuce, tomatoes, carrots, onions, peppers, mushrooms, celery, and cucumbers

2 tablespoons low-fat or fat-free salad dressing

1 serving baked tortilla chips (140 calories per serving)

1,600- & 1,800-CALORIE PLANS

1½ servings chili

Mixed vegetable salad with unlimited lettuce, tomatoes, carrots, onions, peppers, mushrooms, celery, and cucumbers

2 tablespoons low-fat or fat-free salad dressing

1 serving baked tortilla chips (140 calories per serving)

2,000-CALORIE PLAN

2 servings chili

Mixed vegetable salad with unlimited lettuce, tomatoes, carrots, onions, peppers, mushrooms, celery, and cucumbers

2 tablespoons low-fat or fat-free salad dressing

½ serving baked tortilla chips (140 calories per serving), or small toasted whole wheat pita (no more than 70 calories)

Microwave Stuffed Peppers

Serves 4

Choose perfectly shaped green bell peppers for this pretty dish, which has a nicely seasoned filling that's easy to make. Be careful not to overcook the peppers or they won't hold their shape.

4 large peppers (wide for ease)
1 pound extra-lean ground turkey meat
1 envelope dry onion or mushroom-onion soup mix (6 tablespoons dry mix)
1/3 cup water
1/2 cup low-calorie marinara sauce
1/4 cup grated Parmesan cheese

1. Wash the peppers, cut off the tops, and remove the seeds. Place in microwave-safe pan with a cover. Microwave on high for approximately 6 minutes, until the peppers are partially soft but remain firm (do not overcook).

2. In the meantime, brown the turkey meat in a large saucepan. Drain off all fat.

3. In a small bowl, mix the dry soup with the water. Pour the soup mixture over the cooked turkey and stir. Simmer, uncovered, for approximately 10 minutes.

4. Spoon 1/4 of the turkey mixture into each pepper, filling it to the top.

5. Spoon marinara sauce over each pepper (approximately 1 tablespoon on each). Top with 1 tablespoon of Parmesan cheese.

6. Place the peppers in the microwave, cover, and cook on high for 2 minutes. Serve immediately.

◆ **1 SERVING = 1 STUFFED PEPPER**

Calories: 263	Protein: 30 g	Carbohydrates: 15.6 g	Sugar: 0 g	Total fat: 9 g
Saturated fat: 2 g	Cholesterol: 65 mg	Sodium: 1200 mg	Fiber: 3.8 g	Calcium: 132 mg

Vitamin C: 228 mg

1,200-CALORIE PLAN

1 stuffed pepper
Mixed vegetable salad with unlimited lettuce,
  tomatoes, carrots, onions, peppers,
  mushrooms, celery, and cucumbers
2 tablespoons low-fat or fat-free salad
  dressing

1,400-CALORIE PLAN

1 stuffed pepper
Mixed vegetable salad with unlimited lettuce,
  tomatoes, carrots, onions, peppers,
  mushrooms, celery, and cucumbers
2 tablespoons low-fat or fat-free salad
  dressing
1 cup fresh blueberries, 2 cups whole
  strawberries, or 1 apple

1,600- & 1,800-CALORIE PLANS

1 stuffed pepper
Mixed vegetable salad with unlimited lettuce,
  tomatoes, carrots, onions, peppers,
  mushrooms, celery, and cucumbers; $1/4$ cup
  beans (any type); 1 teaspoon Parmesan
  cheese
2 tablespoons low-fat or fat-free salad
  dressing
1 cup fresh blueberries, 2 cups whole
  strawberries, or 1 apple

2,000-CALORIE PLAN

2 stuffed peppers
Mixed vegetable salad with unlimited lettuce,
  tomatoes, carrots, onions, peppers,
  mushrooms, celery, and cucumbers
2 tablespoons low-fat or fat-free salad
  dressing

Portobello Turkey Loaf

Serves 6

My rendition of a classic comfort food tastes extra rich and meaty, thanks to the chopped portobello mushroom and cream of mushroom soup. This is a good recipe to make ahead and freeze in meal-sized portions.

1¾ pounds extra-lean ground turkey breast
1 can low-fat condensed cream of mushroom soup
1 large portobello mushroom, sliced and chopped
Cooking spray

1. Preheat the oven to 350°.

2. In a large bowl, thoroughly mix the turkey meat, mushroom soup, and chopped mushroom.

3. Coat a loaf pan with cooking spray. Add the turkey mixture.

4. Bake for 1½ hours. The turkey loaf will generate a lot of liquid while it cooks. Drain off collected liquid every 30 minutes.

NUTRIENT ANALYSIS

◆ **1 SERVING = 1 SLICE (⅙ LOAF)**

Calories: 217	Protein: 31 g	Carbohydrates: 5.1 g	Sugar: 0.75 g	Total fat: 8 g
Saturated fat: 2 g	Cholesterol: 65 mg	Sodium: 479 mg	Fiber: 1 g	Calcium: 39 mg

1,200-CALORIE PLAN

1 serving turkey loaf

Mixed vegetable salad with unlimited lettuce, tomatoes, carrots, onions, peppers, mushrooms, celery, and cucumbers

2 tablespoons low-fat or fat-free salad dressing

1 cup steamed spinach, broccoli, or Brussels sprouts

1,400-CALORIE PLAN

1½ servings turkey loaf

Mixed vegetable salad with unlimited lettuce, tomatoes, carrots, onions, peppers, mushrooms, celery, and cucumbers

2 tablespoons low-fat or fat-free salad dressing

1 cup steamed spinach, broccoli, Brussels sprouts

1,600- & 1,800-CALORIE PLANS

2 servings turkey loaf

Mixed vegetable salad with unlimited lettuce, tomatoes, carrots, onions, peppers, mushrooms, celery, and cucumbers

2 tablespoons low-fat or fat-free salad dressing

2,000-CALORIE PLAN

2 servings turkey loaf

Mixed vegetable salad with unlimited lettuce, tomatoes, carrots, onions, peppers, mushrooms, celery, and cucumbers, with 2 teaspoons Parmesan cheese

2 tablespoons low-fat or fat-free salad dressing

1 cup steamed spinach, broccoli, or Brussels sprouts

1 teaspoon reduced-fat, soft tub margarine or butter (optional)

Shepherd's Pie with Cauliflower and Turkey

Serves 8

Traditional shepherd's pie contains lamb or mutton mixed with gravy and topped with mashed potatoes. My "unpotato" version is considerably lighter and healthier, and it's packed with vitamins and minerals, thanks to the cauliflower. This recipe is one of my favorites—but it's far from good looking!

2 pounds extra-lean ground turkey breast
2 tablespoons Mrs. Dash
2 tablespoons minced onion
Freshly ground black pepper
2 twenty-ounce bags frozen cauliflower florets
8 ounces nonfat sour cream
8 ounces reduced-fat sour cream
4 tablespoons reduced-fat, soft tub margarine
Salt

1. Preheat the oven to 350°.

2. In a large saucepan, cook the ground turkey, stirring continuously until it is browned and thoroughly cooked. Drain off all fat and season with Mrs. Dash, onion, and pepper. Break up the turkey with a fork so that there aren't any large pieces.

3. Microwave or steam the cauliflower (microwave approximately 8 minutes, then mix through and microwave for another 6 minutes).

4. Mix both sour creams together. Set aside.

5. In a small saucepan, melt the margarine.

6. In a 13" × 9" × 2" baking pan, layer half of the cauliflower on the bottom. Spoon half of the turkey over the cauliflower. Spoon half of the sour cream over the turkey. Carefully spread the sour cream with a spoon evenly over the entire turkey layer. Drizzle half the melted margarine over the sour cream.

7. Repeat, creating a entire second layer of cauliflower, turkey, sour cream, and margarine. Lightly salt the top.

8. Bake, uncovered, for 40 minutes.

NUTRIENT ANALYSIS

♦ 1 SERVING = 1/8 OF CASSEROLE

Calories: 253	Protein: 31 g	Carbohydrates: 11 g	Sugar: 9 g	Total fat: 9.5 g
Saturated fat: 3 g	Cholesterol: 54 mg	Sodium: 324 mg	Fiber: 4 g	Calcium: 105 mg

1,200-CALORIE PLAN

1 serving pie
Mixed vegetable salad with unlimited lettuce, tomatoes, carrots, onions, peppers, mushrooms, celery, and cucumbers
2 tablespoons low-fat or fat-free salad dressing

1,400-CALORIE PLAN

1 serving pie
Mixed vegetable salad with unlimited lettuce, tomatoes, carrots, onions, peppers, mushrooms, celery, and cucumbers
2 tablespoons low-fat or fat-free salad dressing
1 whole pink grapefruit or 1 apple

1,600- & 1,800-CALORIE PLANS

1 1/2 servings pie
Mixed vegetable salad with unlimited lettuce, tomatoes, carrots, onions, peppers, mushrooms, celery, and cucumbers
2 tablespoons low-fat or fat-free salad dressing
1 orange, 1 cup fresh strawberries, or 1/2 pink grapefruit

2,000-CALORIE PLAN

1 1/2 servings pie
Mixed vegetable salad with unlimited lettuce, tomatoes, carrots, onions, peppers, mushrooms, celery, and cucumbers
1/2 cup croutons
2 tablespoons low-fat or fat-free salad dressing
1 orange, 1 cup fresh strawberries, or 1/2 pink grapefruit

Southwestern Turkey Meat Loaf

Serves 6

Forget everything you've ever heard about meat loaf being boring. Chili sauce and cumin give this version a lively flavor, and the chopped vegetables lend an interesting texture.

4 slices firm whole wheat sandwich bread
½ cup chopped onion
½ cup chopped red bell pepper
½ cup packed fresh cilantro sprigs
6 garlic cloves, minced
½ cup + 5 tablespoons bottled chili sauce
1½ pounds extra lean ground turkey
½ cup nonfat sour cream
1 egg
1½ tablespoons Worcestershire sauce
2 teaspoons ground cumin
¾ teaspoon salt
Freshly ground black pepper

1. Preheat the oven to 375°.

2. Tear the bread into pieces. Grind the pieces into fine crumbs in a food processor.

3. In a bowl, combine the onion, pepper, cilantro, and garlic. Stir in ½ cup chili sauce. Add the breadcrumbs and all remaining ingredients and mix well with your hands.

4. Lightly spray a loaf pan with cooking spray. Scoop the meat mixture into the pan and press down firmly to flatten the top. Spread the remaining chili sauce over the top.

5. Bake for 60 to 75 minutes, or until the middle of the loaf registers 170° on a meat thermometer. Allow the meat loaf to cool for 20 minutes before slicing.

◆ **1 SERVING = 1 SLICE (1/6 LOAF)**

Calories: 291	Protein: 30 g	Carbohydrates: 27 g	Sugar: 11 g	Total fat: 7 g

Saturated fat: 2 g	Cholesterol: 90 mg	Sodium: 1,026 mg	Fiber: 1.6 g	Calcium: 86 mg

1,200-CALORIE PLAN

1 serving meat loaf
2 cups mixed green salad
1–2 tablespoons low-fat dressing (or 1
    teaspoon olive oil and 1 tablespoon vinegar)

1,400-CALORIE PLAN

1 serving meat loaf
2 cups mixed green salad
1–2 tablespoons low-fat dressing (or 1
    teaspoon olive oil and 1 tablespoon vinegar)
1 apple; or 1 cup fresh berries, cubed
    pineapple, melon chunks, or grapefruit
    sections

1,600- & 1,800-CALORIE PLANS

1 1/2 servings meat loaf
2 cups mixed green salad
1–2 tablespoons low-fat dressing (or 1
    teaspoon olive oil and 1 tablespoon vinegar)
1 apple; or 1 cup fresh berries, cubed
    pineapple, melon chunks, or grapefruit
    sections

2,000-CALORIE PLAN

1 1/2 servings meat loaf
2 cups mixed green salad topped with 2–3
    tablespoons grated low-fat cheese
2–4 tablespoons low-fat dressing (or 2
    teaspoons olive oil and unlimited vinegar)
1 apple; or 1 cup fresh berries, cubed
    pineapple, melon chunks, or grapefruit
    sections

Tex-Mex Turkey Burgers

Serves 9

If you've got a hankering for a big barbecued burger, try one of these. They're juicy, flavorful, and perfectly seasoned. Adjust the amount of Tabasco up or down depending on your personal taste.

2 pounds extra-lean ground turkey breast
6 tablespoons Stubs Barbecue sauce (or any other brand 30 calories or fewer per tablespoon)
3 tablespoons minced onion flakes (or ½ cup chopped fresh onion)
2 heaping tablespoons Dijon mustard
1 tablespoon Tabasco sauce

1. Combine all the ingredients and mix thoroughly.

2. Divide into 9 patties and grill on a barbecue or under the broiler.

NUTRIENT ANALYSIS

◆ **1 SERVING = 1 PATTY**

Calories: 160	Protein: 24 g	Carbohydrates: 6 g	Sugar: 3.5 g	Total fat: 4 g
Saturated fat: 1.5 g	Cholesterol: 55 mg	Sodium: 261 mg	Fiber: 0 g	Calcium: 19 g

1,200-CALORIE PLAN

1 burger

1 small whole wheat pita (no more than 70 calories)

1 tablespoon catsup

Mixed vegetable salad with unlimited lettuce, tomatoes, carrots, onions, peppers, mushrooms, celery, and cucumbers

2 tablespoons low-fat or fat-free salad dressing

1,400-CALORIE PLAN

1 burger

1 standard hamburger bun, preferably whole wheat

1 slice fat-free sharp cheddar cheese

2 tablespoons catsup

Mixed vegetable salad with unlimited lettuce, tomatoes, carrots, onions, peppers, mushrooms, celery, and cucumbers

2 tablespoons low-fat or fat-free salad dressing

1,600- & 1,800-CALORIE PLANS

1½ burgers

1 standard hamburger bun, preferably whole wheat

1 slice fat-free sharp cheddar cheese

2 tablespoons catsup

Mixed vegetable salad with unlimited lettuce, tomatoes, carrots, onions, peppers, mushrooms, celery, and cucumbers

2 tablespoons low-fat or fat-free salad dressing

2,000-CALORIE PLAN

2 burgers

1 standard hamburger bun, preferably whole wheat

1 slice fat-free sharp cheddar cheese

2 tablespoons catsup

Mixed vegetable salad with unlimited lettuce, tomatoes, carrots, onions, peppers, mushrooms, celery, and cucumbers

2 tablespoons low-fat or fat-free salad dressing

Turkey Loaf with the Kitchen Sink

Serves 6

Everything (or just about everything) goes into this moist, crowd-pleasing meat loaf. It's a great make-ahead dish, too, and you may freeze leftovers for up to a month. If you like, try light beer instead of chicken broth, or low-fat cream of mushroom soup instead of the barbecue sauce. And instead of the broccoli, you can always use portobello mushrooms or chopped spinach.

1¼ to 1½ pounds extra-lean ground turkey breast
2 teaspoons chopped garlic
2 teaspoons Dijon mustard
½ cup barbecue sauce
¼ cup fat-free chicken broth
4 tablespoons grated reduced-fat Parmesan cheese
2 cups fresh broccoli florets, cooked and chopped into small pieces
1 cup cooked corn
1 teaspoon freshly ground black pepper
½ onion, chopped

1. Preheat the oven to 350°.

2. Thoroughly mix all ingredients. Place in a loaf pan and cook, uncovered, for 45 to 60 minutes.

NUTRIENT ANALYSIS

♦ **1 SERVING = 1 SLICE (⅙ LOAF)**

Calories: 220	Protein: 30 g	Carbohydrates: 12.4 g	Sugar: 2.6 g	Total fat: 5 g
Saturated fat: 1.5 g	Cholesterol: 60 mg	Sodium: 300 mg	Fiber: 1.3 g	Calcium: 84 mg

1,200-CALORIE PLAN

1 serving turkey loaf

Mixed vegetable salad with unlimited lettuce, tomatoes, carrots, onions, peppers, mushrooms, celery, and cucumbers

2 tablespoons low-fat or fat-free salad dressing

1 cup steamed cauliflower or green beans

1,400-CALORIE PLAN

1½ servings turkey loaf

Mixed vegetable salad with unlimited lettuce, tomatoes, carrots, onions, peppers, mushrooms, celery, and cucumbers

2 tablespoons low-fat or fat-free salad dressing

1,600- & 1,800-CALORIE PLANS

2 servings turkey loaf

Mixed vegetable salad with unlimited lettuce, tomatoes, carrots, onions, peppers, mushrooms, celery, and cucumbers

2 tablespoons low-fat or fat-free salad dressing

2,000-CALORIE PLAN

2 servings turkey loaf

Mixed vegetable salad with unlimited lettuce, tomatoes, carrots, onions, peppers, mushrooms, celery, cucumbers, and 2 tablespoons corn

3 tablespoons low-fat or fat-free salad dressing

1 cup steamed cauliflower or green beans

Herb-Marinated Flank Steak

Serves 6

This dish features a beautiful presentation: thin slices of herb-crusted, rosy meat are arranged on a plate and garnished with parsley. Thanks to the marinade, it's tender as well as flavorful. To get a head start on your dinner, marinate the meat overnight in the fridge.

½ cup fresh lime juice
1 jalapeño pepper, seeded and chopped
3 cloves garlic, peeled and minced
2 tablespoons chopped fresh mint
2 tablespoons chopped fresh basil
2 tablespoons chopped fresh Italian parsley
2 teaspoons minced fresh ginger
Pinch of salt
1 tablespoon olive oil
1½ pounds flank steak
Additional parsley for garnish

1. In a shallow bowl large enough to hold the flank steak, stir together the lime juice, jalapeño pepper, garlic, mint, basil, parsley, ginger, salt, and olive oil.

2. Score the steak very lightly on both sides. Place it in the marinade. Cover and refrigerate for at least 3 hours or overnight.

3. Remove the steak from the marinade and pat dry with paper towels. Grill the steak on outdoor grill or broiler rack for about 6 minutes per side, or to desired doneness.

4. Allow the steak to rest for 10 minutes. Slice the meat thinly, on the diagonal. Garnish with additional parsley.

◆ 1 SERVING = 3-OUNCE PIECE (SIZE OF A DECK OF CARDS)

Calories: 213	Protein: 25 g	Carbohydrates: 3 g	Sugar: 0 g	Total fat: 10.7 g

Saturated fat: 3.9 g	Cholesterol: 46 mg	Sodium: 169 mg	Fiber: 0.3 g	Calcium: 23 mg

1,200-CALORIE PLAN

1 serving steak

Mixed vegetable salad with unlimited lettuce, tomatoes, carrots, onions, peppers, mushrooms, celery, and cucumbers

2 tablespoons low-fat or fat-free salad dressing

1 cup steamed broccoli

1 teaspoon melted reduced-fat, soft tub margarine or butter (optional)

1,400-CALORIE PLAN

1 1/2 servings steak

Mixed vegetable salad with unlimited lettuce, tomatoes, carrots, onions, peppers, mushrooms, celery, and cucumbers

2 tablespoons low-fat or fat-free salad dressing

1 cup steamed broccoli

1 teaspoon melted reduced-fat, soft tub margarine or butter (optional)

1,600- & 1,800-CALORIE PLANS

2 servings steak

Mixed vegetable salad with unlimited lettuce, tomatoes, carrots, onions, peppers, mushrooms, celery, and cucumbers

2 tablespoons low-fat or fat-free salad dressing

1 cup steamed broccoli

1 teaspoon melted reduced-fat, soft tub margarine or butter (optional)

2,000-CALORIE PLAN

2 servings steak

Mixed vegetable salad with unlimited lettuce, tomatoes, carrots, onions, peppers, mushrooms, celery, and cucumbers

2 tablespoons low-fat or fat-free salad dressing

1 cup steamed broccoli

1 teaspoon melted reduced-fat, soft tub margarine or butter (optional)

Small toasted whole wheat pita (no more than 70 calories)

Slow-Cooker Beef Stroganoff

Serves 6

Start this savory stew before you leave the house, and by dinnertime, the meat will be cooked to perfect tenderness. Served over egg noodles and garnished with fat-free sour cream, it's a meat lover's dream.

1½ pounds boneless beef round steak, trimmed of any visible fat and cut into ¼-inch slices
1 onion, peeled and thinly sliced
2 cloves garlic, crushed
1½ tablespoons Worcestershire sauce
Freshly ground black pepper
½ teaspoon salt
¾ teaspoon paprika
1¼ cups canned beef broth
2½ tablespoons catsup
1½ tablespoons red wine
3 tablespoons cornstarch
¼ cup cold water
½ pound button mushrooms, stems removed, sliced
½ cup fat-free sour cream
3 cups cooked egg noodles

1. In a large (3- or 3½-quart) slow cooker, combine the steak, onion, garlic, Worcestershire sauce, pepper, salt, paprika, beef broth, catsup, and wine. Stir well. Cover and cook on low for 7 hours, or until the steak is tender.

2. In a small bowl, dissolve the cornstarch in the water. Add to the slow cooker, along with the mushrooms. Replace the cover and cook on high for 20 minutes, or until the sauce is bubbling hot. Stir in the sour cream and serve over the noodles.

◆ **1 SERVING = ⅙ OF STEW**

Calories: 382	Protein: 41 g	Carbohydrates: 30.5 g	Sugar: 4.3 g	Total fat: 9.9 g

Saturated fat: 3.7 g	Cholesterol: 106.7 mg	Sodium: 549 mg	Fiber: 1.7 g	Calcium: 72 mg

1,200-CALORIE PLAN

1 serving Beef Stroganoff

Chopped lettuce with 2 teaspoons balsamic vinegar

1,400-CALORIE PLAN

1 serving Beef Stroganoff

Chopped lettuce with 2 teaspoons balsamic vinegar and 1 teaspoon olive oil

1 cup steamed sugar snap peas, cauliflower, carrots, or zucchini

1,600- & 1,800-CALORIE PLANS

1 serving Beef Stroganoff

Chopped lettuce and tomato with 2 teaspoons balsamic vinegar and 1 teaspoon olive oil

1½ cups steamed sugar snap peas, cauliflower, carrots, or zucchini

1 teaspoon reduced-fat, soft tub margarine or butter (optional)

2,000-CALORIE PLAN

1½ servings Beef Stroganoff

1½ cups steamed sugar snap peas, cauliflower, carrots, or zucchini

1 teaspoon reduced-fat, soft tub margarine or butter (optional)

Pork Lo Mein

Serves 6

If you love ordering lo mein in a Chinese restaurant, try this lightened version of a beloved classic. Soy sauce and apple juice replace some of the oil, and there are plenty of colorful, crunchy vegetables along with the meat and noodles.

1½ tablespoons cornstarch
2 tablespoons low-sodium soy sauce
2 tablespoons apple juice
Cooking spray
1 pound boneless pork loin, all visible fat removed, cut into julienne strips
Salt
1 pound egg noodles
3 tablespoons vegetable oil
1 teaspoon minced fresh ginger
2 garlic cloves, peeled and chopped
1 cup cauliflower florets
1 red bell pepper, cored, seeded, and cut into thin strips
2 cups snow peas
½ cup sliced mushrooms
1 zucchini, ends removed, sliced into half moons
1 yellow summer squash, ends removed, sliced into half moons
1 teaspoon sugar
1 can fat-free chicken broth

1. In a small glass measuring cup, stir the cornstarch, soy sauce, and apple juice.

2. Heat a large nonstick skillet. Spray lightly with cooking spray. Stir-fry the pork strips for 4 to 5 minutes, until done. Remove the meat from the pan and sprinkle with a little salt. Wipe the pan clean with a paper towel.

3. In a large pot of boiling salted water, cook the noodles according to package directions. Drain and set aside.

4. Heat 1 tablespoon of the oil in the skillet. Add the noodles and stir-fry for 4 minutes. Remove the noodles to a bowl and cover loosely with foil.

5. Heat the remaining 2 tablespoons of oil in the skillet and add the ginger, garlic, and cauliflower. Stir-fry for 3 minutes. Add the remaining vegetables and stir-fry for 2 minutes. Sprinkle with sugar. Pour in the broth and bring to a boil. Add the reserved cornstarch mixture. Add the cooked pork strips and stir until the sauce is thick.

6. Mix the meat mixture with the noodles and stir gently to combine.

NUTRIENT ANALYSIS

◆ **1 SERVING = 2 CUPS**

Calories: 319	Protein: 23 g	Carbohydrates: 28.4 g	Sugar: 4.8 g	Total fat: 12.3 g
Saturated fat: 2.6 g	Cholesterol: 72.5 mg	Sodium: 403 mg	Fiber: 3 g	Calcium: 54 mg

1,200-CALORIE PLAN

1 serving lo mein
Chopped lettuce, cucumber, and onion salad
1 tablespoon low-fat or fat-free salad dressing

1,400-CALORIE PLAN

1 serving lo mein
Chopped lettuce, cucumber, and onion salad
2 tablespoons low-fat or fat-free salad dressing
1 apple or 2 cups whole strawberries

1,600- & 1,800-CALORIE PLANS

1½ servings lo mein (3 cups)
Chopped lettuce, cucumber, and onion salad
2 tablespoons low-fat or fat-free salad dressing

2,000-CALORIE PLAN

1½ servings lo mein (3 cups)
Chopped lettuce, cucumber, and onion salad
3 tablespoons low-fat or fat-free salad dressing
1 apple or 2 cups whole strawberries

Asian Citrus Salmon Steak

Serves 4

This recipe was one of the favorites at ABC's Good Morning America's *"Lock the Door, Lose the Weight" segment series. For maximum flavor, start marinating the steaks several hours before you plan to cook dinner. You'll be rewarded with moist, succulent salmon accented with just the right balance of orange, garlic, and soy sauce.*

½ cup low-sodium soy sauce
¼ cup orange juice
2 tablespoons chopped garlic
2 teaspoons mustard
2 teaspoons tomato sauce or marinara sauce
Juice of ½ lemon
4 six-ounce salmon steaks

1. In a bowl, mix all the ingredients except the salmon. Pour the mixture, along with the salmon, into a large ziplock bag.

2. Seal the bag and squish it with your hands until the salmon is coated with the marinade. Refrigerate for 4 to 6 hours

3. Place the salmon steaks on a grill for approximately 5 minutes on each side (or longer for well done). You may also use an oven broiler—broil for 3 to 5 minutes per side.

NUTRIENT ANALYSIS

◆ **1 SERVING = 1 STEAK**

Calories: 277	Protein: 36 g	Carbohydrates: 7.5 g	Sugar: 5.1 g	Total fat: 10.9 g
Saturated fat: 1.6 g	Cholesterol: 93 mg	Sodium: 1319 mg	Fiber: 1.1 g	Calcium: 44 mg

1,200-CALORIE PLAN

1 serving salmon

2 cups raw spinach sautéed in 1 teaspoon olive oil and garlic

1,400-CALORIE PLAN

1 serving salmon

Mixed vegetable salad with unlimited lettuce, tomatoes, carrots, onions, peppers, mushrooms, celery, and cucumbers

2 tablespoons low-fat or fat-free salad dressing

2 cups raw spinach sautéed in 1 teaspoon olive oil and garlic

1,600- & 1,800-CALORIE PLANS

1 serving salmon

Mixed vegetable salad with unlimited lettuce, tomatoes, carrots, onions, peppers, mushrooms, celery, and cucumbers

2 tablespoons low-fat or fat-free salad dressing

2 cups raw spinach sautéed in 1 teaspoon olive oil and garlic

$1/2$ cup cooked couscous or brown rice

2,000-CALORIE PLAN

1 serving salmon

Mixed vegetable salad with unlimited lettuce, tomatoes, carrots, onions, peppers, mushrooms, celery, and cucumbers

2 tablespoons low-fat or fat-free salad dressing

2 cups raw spinach sautéed in 1 teaspoon olive oil and garlic

1 cup cooked couscous or brown rice

Honey Mustard Salmon

Serves 4

Honey and mustard are natural to offset the rich flavor of salmon, which in this entrée is lightly grilled to perfection. If you don't have a barbecue, use the oven broiler instead.

5 tablespoons honey mustard
2 tablespoons low-sodium soy sauce
2 teaspoons chopped garlic
4 six-ounce salmon steak fillets
Salt and freshly ground black pepper

1. In a bowl, mix together the mustard, soy sauce, and garlic.

2. Cover both sides of the salmon with the mixture.

3. Place the salmon on the barbecue. Grill on both sides until pink and tender.

4. Add salt and pepper to taste.

NUTRIENT ANALYSIS

◆ **1 SERVING = 1 FILLET**

Calories: 282	Protein: 34.4 g	Carbohydrates: 6.75 g	Sugar: 5.7 g	Total fat: 10.75 g
Saturated fat: 1.6 g	Cholesterol: 93.5 mg	Sodium: 575 mg	Fiber: 0 g	Calcium: 27 mg

1,200-CALORIE PLAN

1 serving salmon

Mixed vegetable salad with unlimited lettuce,
tomatoes, carrots, onions, peppers,
mushrooms, celery, and cucumbers

2 tablespoons low-fat or fat-free salad
dressing

1,400-CALORIE PLAN

1 serving salmon

Mixed vegetable salad with unlimited lettuce,
tomatoes, carrots, onions, peppers,
mushrooms, celery, and cucumbers

2 tablespoons low-fat or fat-free salad
dressing

1/2 medium (7-ounce) baked potato, plain

1,600- & 1,800-CALORIE PLANS

1 serving salmon

Mixed vegetable salad with unlimited lettuce,
tomatoes, carrots, onions, peppers,
mushrooms, celery, and cucumbers

2 tablespoons low-fat or fat-free salad
dressing

1 medium (7-ounce) baked potato, plain

2,000-CALORIE PLAN

1 serving salmon

Mixed vegetable salad with unlimited lettuce,
tomatoes, carrots, onions, peppers,
mushrooms, celery, and cucumbers

2 tablespoons low-fat or fat-free salad
dressing

1 medium (7-ounce) baked potato

1 teaspoon reduced-fat, soft tub margarine or
butter

1 tablespoon reduced-fat sour cream

Maple-Glazed Salmon

Serves 4

A lightly sweetened, ginger-scented marinade enriches the flavor of this salmon dish, which is a perfect candidate for cooking on a stovetop grill. Don't leave the salmon in the marinade for more than a couple of hours or it might become mushy.

2 tablespoons maple syrup
1½ tablespoons grated fresh ginger
Dash of cayenne pepper
¼ cup orange juice
¼ cup sherry
¼ cup low-sodium soy sauce
¼ cup Dijon mustard
4 six-ounce salmon fillets
Cooking spray
4 scallions, washed and trimmed
1 lemon, quartered

1. In a large, shallow bowl, stir together the maple syrup, ginger, cayenne pepper, orange juice, sherry, soy sauce, and mustard. Place the salmon fillets in the marinade. Cover and refrigerate for 40 minutes or up to 1½ hours.

2. Spray a heavy stovetop grill pan with cooking spray. Heat over medium-high heat. Dry the salmon fillets with paper towel and reserve the marinade.

3. Place the salmon fillets on the hot grill pan and cook for 3 to 5 minutes on each side. Meanwhile, boil the marinade briskly for 1 minute. Baste the salmon several times with the reserved marinade.

4. When the fish flakes easily with a fork, remove it from the pan. Garnish each serving with a scallion and a wedge of lemon.

◆ **1 SERVING = 1 FILLET**

Calories: 337	Protein: 36.5 g	Carbohydrates: 17 g	Sugar: 11 g	Total fat: 12 g
Saturated fat: 1.7 g	Cholesterol: 94 mg	Sodium: 765 mg	Fiber: 2.2 g	Calcium: 81 mg

1,200-CALORIE PLAN

1 salmon fillet

1 cup steamed mushrooms, green beans, or broccoli

1,400-CALORIE PLAN

1 salmon fillet

1 cup steamed mushrooms, green beans, or broccoli

1/2 cup cooked brown rice

1,600- & 1,800-CALORIE PLANS

1 salmon fillet

1 cup steamed mushrooms, green beans, or broccoli

3/4 cup cooked brown rice

2,000-CALORIE PLAN

1 salmon fillet

1 cup mushrooms, green beans, or broccoli sautéed in 1 teaspoon olive oil and garlic

1 cup cooked brown rice

Lemon Pepper–Seared Tuna Steaks

Serves 4

What could be simpler or more delicious than a four-ingredient fresh tuna entrée? This one gets its lovely taste from fresh lemon juice and cilantro. An alternative to the oven broiler is to cook this outside on your barbecue grill.

2 fresh lemons
4 six-ounce tuna steaks
Lemon-pepper seasoning
½ cup fresh chopped cilantro

1. Squeeze the lemon juice onto the tuna. Coat all sides with the lemon-pepper seasoning.

2. Place the tuna under the broiler. Cook for 4 to 5 minutes on each side.

3. Sprinkle with chopped cilantro.

NUTRIENT ANALYSIS

◆ **1 SERVING = 1 STEAK**

Calories: 271	Protein: 42 g	Carbohydrates: 6.8 g	Sugar: 1.3 g	Total fat: 8.9 g
Saturated fat: 2.2 g	Cholesterol: 67 mg	Sodium: 221 mg	Fiber: 3 g	Calcium: 58 mg

1,200-CALORIE PLAN

1 tuna steak
1 cup steamed zucchini
$1/2$ grapefruit or orange

1,400-CALORIE PLAN

1 tuna steak
1 cup steamed zucchini
1 teaspoon melted reduced-fat, soft tub
  margarine or butter
$1/2$ baked medium sweet potato, plain

1,600- & 1,800-CALORIE PLANS

1 tuna steak
1 cup steamed zucchini
1 baked medium sweet potato, plain

2,000-CALORIE PLAN

1 tuna steak
1 cup steamed zucchini
1 baked medium sweet potato, plain
1 teaspoon reduced-fat, soft tub margarine or
  butter
1 apple, 2 cups whole strawberries, or 1 cup
  cubed pineapple

Shrimp with Garlic and Feta

Serves 6

Tangy feta cheese and an infusion of fresh garlic enliven this variation on the classic scampi. It's served over brown rice, which is a good source of fiber and has a chewy, pleasantly nutty flavor. Be sure to halve the amount of feta if you're following the 1,200-calorie plan.

1 tablespoon olive oil
6 garlic cloves, minced
2 twenty-eight-ounce cans whole tomatoes, drained and chopped
½ cup chopped fresh parsley
1½ pounds large shrimp, peeled and deveined
1¼ cups crumbled feta cheese (for 1,200-calorie plan, use just under ⅔ cup)
2 tablespoons freshly squeezed lemon juice
Freshly ground black pepper
3 cups cooked brown rice

1. Preheat the oven to 400°.

2. In a large flameproof casserole, heat the oil over medium heat. Add the garlic and sauté for 30 seconds. Add the tomatoes and half the parsley. Reduce the heat and simmer for 12 minutes.

3. Stir in the shrimp. Cook over medium heat for 5 minutes.

4. Pour the mixture into a 13" × 9" baking dish and sprinkle with the feta. Bake for 10 minutes.

5. Just before serving, sprinkle with the remaining parsley, lemon juice, and pepper.

NUTRIENT ANALYSIS

◆ 1 SERVING = ⅙ OF SHRIMP ENTRÉE

Calories: 380	Protein: 33 g	Carbohydrates: 34 g	Sugar: 6.3 g	Total fat: 12 g
Saturated fat: 5.5 g	Cholesterol: 200 mg	Sodium: 1247 mg	Fiber: 3.1 g	Calcium: 297 mg

1,200-CALORIE PLAN

1 serving shrimp
$^1/_2$ cup cooked brown rice

1,400-CALORIE PLAN

1 serving shrimp
$^1/_2$ cup cooked brown rice
1 cup steamed broccoli

1,600- & 1,800-CALORIE PLANS

1 serving shrimp
1 cup cooked brown rice
1 cup steamed broccoli

2,000-CALORIE PLAN

1$^1/_2$ servings shrimp
1 cup cooked brown rice
1 cup steamed broccoli

Spicy Jambalaya

Serves 6

A Creole specialty that'll make you feel like you're dining in New Orleans, this is a stick-to-the-ribs dish that boasts shrimp, turkey sausage, and chicken breast. Adjust the cayenne pepper according to how much heat you like in your food. If you're following the 1,200-calorie plan, be sure to remove your portion before adding the rice to the pot.

Cooking spray
2 teaspoons olive oil
1 medium onion, peeled and chopped
2 ribs celery, no leaves, chopped
½ green pepper, seeded, cored, and chopped
2 tablespoons tomato paste
1½ teaspoons dried basil
¼ teaspoon cayenne pepper
1 teaspoon salt
3 garlic cloves, peeled and chopped
½ pound turkey sausage, sliced
½ pound boneless chicken breast, cut into large cubes
2 cans (14.5 ounces each) stewed tomatoes prepared
  with garlic and pepper
2 ounces diced pimiento, well drained
2 bay leaves
3 cups *cooked* white rice
½ pound medium shrimp, peeled and deveined
  (thawed if frozen)

1. Spray a large heavy nonstick skillet with cooking spray. Add the olive oil, onion, celery, and green pepper. Cook over medium-high heat, stirring, for 5 minutes.

2. Stir in the tomato paste, basil, cayenne pepper, salt, garlic, turkey sausage, and chicken. Cook for 5 minutes, stirring. Add the stewed tomatoes, pimiento, and bay leaves and cook for another 5 minutes, or until the meat is thoroughly cooked.

3. Remove the bay leaves. Stir in the rice* and the shrimp and cook for another 5 minutes, or until the shrimp is cooked and the jambalaya is thoroughly hot.

*If you are following the 1,200-calorie plan, eat the jambalaya without rice. Remove 1 serving (1 cup) after the shrimp is cooked, then add the rice.

NUTRIENT ANALYSIS

- **1 SERVING = 1 CUP, NO RICE (1,200 CALORIE PLAN)**
- **1 SERVING = 1¼ CUP (ALL OTHER PLANS) ANALYSIS DONE FOR THIS VERSION**

Calories: 420	Protein: 26.5 g	Carbohydrates: 38.8 g	Sugar: 6.6 g	Total fat: 17.8 g
Saturated fat: 4.5 g	Cholesterol: 108 mg	Sodium: 1,129 mg	Fiber: 2.6 g	Calcium: 107 mg

1,200-CALORIE PLAN

1 serving jambalaya (without rice)
1 cup steamed mushrooms, or 1 sliced cucumber

1,400-CALORIE PLAN

1 serving jambalaya
1 cup steamed mushrooms, or 1 sliced cucumber

1,600- & 1,800-CALORIE PLANS

1 serving jambalaya
Mixed vegetable salad with unlimited lettuce, tomatoes, carrots, onions, peppers, mushrooms, celery, and cucumbers
2 tablespoons low-fat or fat-free salad dressing
1 cup steamed mushrooms or carrots
1 teaspoon melted reduced-fat, soft tub margarine or butter (optional)

2,000-CALORIE PLAN

1½ servings jambalaya
1 cup steamed mushrooms, or 1 sliced cucumber

Angel Hair Pasta Piccata

Serves 4

Piccata usually refers to chicken or veal that's sautéed and served with a lemon and parsley sauce. This vegetarian version is light and lemony, and it's flavored with a generous helping of fresh basil as well as parsley.

1 tablespoon olive oil
3 garlic cloves, peeled and chopped
2 scallions, white part only, chopped
1/2 cup dry white wine
Juice of 1 large lemon
1/8 teaspoon ground white pepper
1 tomato, seeded and chopped
1/2 pound angel hair pasta
1/4 cup chopped fresh basil
3 tablespoons freshly grated Parmesan cheese
1 tablespoon chopped fresh parsley

1. In a sauté pan, heat the oil over medium heat. Add the garlic and scallions and cook for 2 minutes, or until the garlic is golden. Remove the pan from the heat.

2. Add the wine to the pan and simmer for 3 minutes, or until the wine is reduced by half. Add the lemon juice, white pepper, and tomato. Stir well and remove the pan from the heat.

3. Cook the pasta in a large pot of boiling, salted water for 1 minute or until al dente. Drain the pasta and place it into a serving bowl. Toss it with the tomato mixture, fresh basil, and Parmesan cheese. Garnish with chopped parsley.

NUTRIENT ANALYSIS

♦ **1 SERVING = 1 CUP**

Calories: 252	Protein: 9.3 g	Carbohydrates: 35 g	Sugar: 2.3 g	Total fat: 6.7 g
Saturated fat: 1.9 g	Cholesterol: 66.7 mg	Sodium: 266 mg	Fiber: 2.2 g	Calcium: 85.7 mg

1,200-CALORIE PLAN

1 serving pasta

Mixed vegetable salad with unlimited lettuce,
tomatoes, carrots, onions, peppers,
mushrooms, celery, and cucumbers

2 tablespoons low-fat or fat-free salad
dressing

1,400-CALORIE PLAN

$1^1/_2$ servings pasta

Mixed vegetable salad with unlimited lettuce,
tomatoes, carrots, onions, peppers,
mushrooms, celery, and cucumbers

2 tablespoons low-fat or fat-free salad
dressing

1,600- & 1,800-CALORIE PLANS

$1^1/_2$ servings pasta

Mixed vegetable salad with unlimited lettuce,
tomatoes, carrots, onions, peppers,
mushrooms, celery, and cucumbers

2 tablespoons low-fat or fat-free salad
dressing

$^1/_4$ cantaloupe, 1 whole grapefruit, 1 apple, or
1 cup cubed pineapple

2,000-CALORIE PLAN

2 servings pasta

Mixed vegetable salad with unlimited lettuce,
tomatoes, carrots, onions, peppers,
mushrooms, celery, and cucumbers

2 tablespoons low-fat or fat-free salad
dressing

$^1/_4$ cantaloupe, 1 whole grapefruit, 1 apple, or
1 cup cubed pineapple

Cold Sesame Noodles

Serves 6

Typically, sesame noodles are incredibly high in fat, thanks to the oil and the peanut butter. While these are lightened with lime juice, unsweetened applesauce, and skim milk, they retain the nutty richness and satisfying crunch that make this dish so popular. Plus, this version is high in fiber—6 grams per 1-cup serving.

3 tablespoons peanut butter
1½ teaspoons lime juice
2 tablespoons natural applesauce (unsweetened)
1 tablespoon low-sodium soy sauce
2 tablespoons skim milk
8 ounces whole wheat pasta
2 tablespoons sesame oil
5 tablespoons sesame seeds

1. In a bowl, mix the peanut butter, lime juice, applesauce, soy sauce, and skim milk. Stir until well blended.

2. Cook the pasta as directed.

3. Pour the entire peanut butter mixture over the cooked pasta and gently but thoroughly mix. Add the sesame oil and mix.

4. Sprinkle 2 tablespoons of sesame seeds over the pasta and toss. Repeat with the remaining 3 tablespoons of seeds. Sesame seeds should be evenly scattered throughout the pasta.

5. Serve at room temperature or slightly chilled.

◆ **1 SERVING = 1 CUP**

| Calories: 251 | Protein: 7.8 g | Carbohydrates: 32 g | Sugar: 2.9 g | Total fat: 11.2 g |

| Saturated fat: 1.8 g | Cholesterol: 0 mg | Sodium: 224 mg | Fiber: 6 g | Calcium: 46 mg |

1,200-CALORIE PLAN

1 serving noodles
¾ cup boiled soybeans in the pod
  (edamame), lightly salted
Or
1 serving noodles
Salad of lettuce and cucumbers
2 tablespoons low-fat or fat-free dressing
1 cup steamed spinach topped with
  1–2 teaspoons low-sodium soy sauce

1,400-CALORIE PLAN

1½ servings noodles
¾ cup boiled soybeans in the pod
  (edamame), lightly salted
Or
1½ servings noodles
Salad of lettuce and cucumbers
2 tablespoons low-fat or fat-free dressing
1 cup steamed spinach topped with
  1–2 teaspoons low-sodium soy sauce

1,600- & 1,800-CALORIE PLANS

2 servings noodles
½ cup boiled soybeans in the pod
  (edamame), lightly salted
Or
2 servings noodles
1 cup steamed spinach topped with
  1–2 teaspoons low-sodium soy sauce

2,000-CALORIE PLAN

2 servings noodles
1 cup boiled soybeans in the pod (edamame),
  lightly salted
Or
2½ servings noodles
1 cup steamed spinach topped with
  1–2 teaspoons low-sodium soy sauce

Baked Cauliflower Puree

Serves 6

Creamy and rich-tasting, this is real comfort food. Add a piece of grilled chicken or a plain turkey burger, and you've got a great, easy meal.

2 twenty ounce bags frozen cauliflower florets (or 14 cups fresh cauliflower florets)
1 cup (8 ounces) reduced-fat sour cream
2 tablespoons reduced-fat, soft tub margarine
1/4 teaspoon salt
1/4 cup breadcrumbs (garlic and herb flavor)
2 tablespoons grated reduced-fat Parmesan cheese
add freshly ground pepper to taste

1. Preheat the oven to 350°.

2. Place the cauliflower in a large microwave-safe dish, cover with a paper towel, and microwave on high for 10 minutes. Remove from the microwave, stir up the cauliflower, and microwave for another 10 minutes. The cauliflower should be soft and mushy.

3. To the cauliflower, add the sour cream, margarine, and salt, and puree with a hand mixer.

4. Spread the cauliflower puree evenly into a 12" × 9" × 1¼" baking pan.

5. Mix together the breadcrumbs and Parmesan cheese. Sprinkle evenly over the cauliflower puree.

6. Bake 1 hour and 15 minutes (breadcrumbs will become slightly browned).

7. Let cool and cut into 6 servings.

NUTRIENT ANALYSIS

♦ 1 SERVING = ⅙ OF PUREE

Calories: 135   Protein: 6 g   Carbohydrates: 14 g   Sugar: 0 g   Total fat: 7 g

Saturated fat: 3.5 g   Cholesterol: 15.8 mg   Sodium: 287 mg   Fiber: 4.5 g   Calcium: 111 mg

1,200-CALORIE PLAN

1 serving cauliflower
1 Tex-Mex Turkey Burger (see recipe on page 149)
$1/2$ sliced tomato

1,400-CALORIE PLAN

1 serving cauliflower
1 Tex-Mex Turkey Burger (see recipe on page 149)
$1/2$ sliced tomato
2 tablespoons catsup or barbecue sauce
$1/2$ standard hamburger bun (preferably whole wheat)

1,600- & 1,800-CALORIE PLANS

1 serving cauliflower
1 Tex-Mex Turkey Burger (see recipe on page 149)
$1/2$ sliced tomato
2 tablespoons catsup or barbecue sauce
1 standard hamburger bun (preferably whole wheat)

2,000-CALORIE PLAN

2 servings cauliflower
1 Tex-Mex Turkey Burger (see recipe on page 149)
$1/2$ sliced tomato
2 tablespoons catsup or barbecue sauce
1 standard hamburger bun (preferably whole wheat)

Spinach-Cheese Timbale

Serves 2

This recipe yields two very generous servings, and the dish is elegant enough to serve to company. If you prefer, substitute frozen chopped broccoli for the spinach.

1 cup 1% low-fat cottage cheese
1/2 cup plain nonfat yogurt
1/3 cup crumbled feta cheese
1/4 teaspoon salt
1/2 teaspoon dried basil
Freshly ground black pepper
2 eggs
2 egg whites
1 ten-ounce package frozen chopped spinach, thawed and drained, as much water as possible removed

1. Preheat the oven to 350°.

2. In a large mixing bowl, combine the cottage cheese, yogurt, feta, salt, basil, pepper, eggs, and egg whites. Beat with electric mixer until blended. Add the spinach and mix thoroughly with a spoon.

3. Place the mixture into a 1-quart casserole dish and bake for 1½ hours, or until a knife inserted near the center comes out clean. Place on rack to cool briefly.

NUTRIENT ANALYSIS

♦ 1 SERVING = ½ OF TIMBALE

Calories: 310	Protein: 34 g	Carbohydrates: 14 g	Sugar: 7 g	Total fat: 12 g
Saturated fat: 6 g	Cholesterol: 98 mg	Sodium: 1387 mg	Fiber: 4 g	Calcium: 450 mg

1,200-CALORIE PLAN

1 serving timbale

1 sliced cucumber

1,400-CALORIE PLAN

1 serving timbale

1/2 medium baked or sweet potato, plain

1,600- & 1,800-CALORIE PLANS

1 serving timbale

1 medium baked or sweet potato, plain

2,000-CALORIE PLAN

2 servings timbale

Or

1 serving spinach

1 medium baked or sweet potato

2 tablespoons reduced-fat sour cream or
   1 tablespoon light butter spread

1 orange, 1/2 grapefruit, or 1 cup strawberries

Vegetable and White Bean Salad

Serves 4

Canned beans are one of the best convenience foods to keep on hand, because you can save yourself hours of time on soaking and cooking dried beans when you want a fast, protein-rich lunch. This colorful, crunchy salad can be assembled two hours ahead of time. Just before serving, line plates with curly endive and scoop a portion of salad into the center of each plate.

3 carrots, peeled and diced
3 tablespoons balsamic vinegar
2 tablespoons olive oil
Pinch of salt
1/4 teaspoon dried basil
Pinch of dried thyme
Pinch of dried sage
Freshly ground black pepper
3 garlic cloves, peeled and minced
1 large yellow bell pepper, chopped
1/2 cup sliced scallions
1 dozen cherry tomatoes, quartered
1 sixteen-ounce can cannellini beans, rinsed and drained
4 cups curly endive, washed and dried

1. Cook the carrots in water for 1 minute. Rinse and drain.

2. In large bowl, combine the vinegar, oil, salt, basil, thyme, sage, and pepper. Stir well. Stir in the carrots, garlic, bell pepper, scallions, tomatoes, and cannellini beans. Toss gently to combine.

3. Line 4 chilled plates with the endive. Spoon the salad onto the endive and serve.

◆ **1 SERVING = APPROXIMATELY 1½ CUPS**

Calories: 293	Protein: 13 g	Carbohydrates: 45 g	Sugar: 6.3 g	Total fat: 7.6
Saturated fat: 1 g	Cholesterol: 0 mg	Sodium: 162 mg	Fiber: 11.5 g	Calcium: 167 mg

1,200-CALORIE PLAN

1 serving salad

1 small whole wheat pita (70 calories),
5 saltines, or 1 cup berries

1,400-CALORIE PLAN

1 serving salad

1 regular-size whole wheat pita (no more than
150 calories) or 1 serving reduced-fat Wheat
Thins (approximately 16 crackers)

1,600- & 1,800-CALORIE PLANS

1 serving salad

1 regular-size whole wheat pita (no more than
150 calories) or 1 serving reduced-fat Wheat
Thins (approximately 16 crackers)

1 apple or 1 pear; 1 cup berries, cubed
pineapple, or melon chunks; ½ mango; or
1 small banana

2,000-CALORIE PLAN

1 serving salad

1 regular-size whole wheat pita (no more than
150 calories) or 1 serving reduced-fat Wheat
Thins (approximately 16 crackers)

1 apple or 1 pear; 1 cup berries, cubed
pineapple, or melon chunks; ½ mango; or
½ banana

8 ounces nonfat flavored yogurt (any brand
that is 120 calories or fewer per 8 ounces)

Black Bean Soup with Sherry and Garlic

Serves 8 (2 cup servings)

Soup lovers will enjoy this thick, nourishing, perfectly seasoned version of a classic. It freezes very well; divide it into serving-sized portions and defrost when you need an easy supper on a cold winter night.

1 pound dried black beans
Cooking spray
1 tablespoon olive oil
2 medium onions, peeled and chopped
2 carrots, peeled and chopped
3 stalks celery, no leaves, tough ends discarded, chopped
1 green bell pepper, seeded, cored, and chopped
1 red bell pepper, seeded, cored, and chopped
3 garlic cloves, peeled and minced
¾ cup dry sherry
2 tablespoons ground cumin
1½ tablespoons chili powder
¾ tablespoon dried oregano
1 tablespoon honey
1 tablespoon Splenda
¼ teaspoon ground cinnamon
½ teaspoon ground chipotle chili
2 bay leaves
Dash of freshly ground black pepper
½ teaspoon sea salt
1 large can (49 ounces) fat-free chicken broth
2 cans (14.5 ounces) diced tomatoes, drained
8 tablespoons fat-free sour cream
8 sprigs fresh cilantro

1. Sort and rinse the beans. Discard any that are discolored. Place the beans in a large Dutch oven. Cover with about 4 cups of water; the water level should be 1½ inches above the beans. Bring to a boil and cook for 3 minutes. Cover and let the beans stand for an hour.

2. Drain the beans and add 4 cups more water. Bring to a boil, cover, reduce the heat, and cook for 1 hour, or until the beans are soft. Drain the beans and set them aside.

3. Meanwhile, spray a large, heavy nonstick sauté pan with cooking spray. Add the olive oil, onions, carrots, celery, peppers, and garlic. Sauté over medium heat for 8 minutes. Add the cooked beans, sherry, cumin, chili powder, oregano, honey, Splenda, cinnamon, chipotle chili, bay leaves, pepper, and sea salt. Stir well. Add the chicken broth and diced tomatoes and stir again. Simmer, covered, for 30 minutes. Discard the bay leaves.

4. Use a slotted spoon to measure out 4 cups of the bean mixture. Puree the remaining soup in a blender in several batches. Return the pureed soup and the bean mixture to the sauté pan and simmer for 10 minutes, or until thoroughly heated.

5. Ladle the soup into 8 bowls and top each bowl with 1 tablespoon fat-free sour cream and a cilantro sprig.

NUTRIENT ANALYSIS

◆ **1 SERVING = 2 CUPS SOUP WITH 1 TABLESPOON NONFAT SOUR CREAM**

Calories: 332	Protein: 16.5 g	Carbohydrates: 54 g	Sugar: 11 g	Total fat: 3.2 g
Saturated fat: 0.5 g	Cholesterol: 1.4 mg	Sodium: 271 mg	Fiber: 12.6 g	Calcium: 185 mg

1,200-CALORIE PLAN

1 serving soup

1,400-CALORIE PLAN

1 serving soup

Mixed vegetable salad with unlimited lettuce, tomatoes, carrots, onions, peppers, mushrooms, celery, and cucumbers

2 tablespoons low-fat or fat-free salad dressing

1 orange or 1 cup strawberries

1,600- & 1,800-CALORIE PLANS

1 serving soup

Mixed vegetable salad with unlimited lettuce, tomatoes, carrots, onions, peppers, mushrooms, celery, and cucumbers

2 tablespoons low-fat or fat-free salad dressing

1 serving baked tortilla chips (140 calories or fewer per serving)

2,000-CALORIE PLAN

1 serving soup

Mixed vegetable salad with unlimited lettuce, tomatoes, carrots, onions, peppers, mushrooms, celery, and cucumbers

2 tablespoons low-fat or fat-free salad dressing

1 serving baked tortilla chips (140 calories or fewer per serving)

$1/2$ cup shredded low-fat cheddar cheese to melt on tortilla chips

Seven

Gourmet Dinners and Festive Holiday Menus

Ground Sirloin Steak Smothered in Caramelized Onions
    Smashed Yukon Gold Potatoes with Buttermilk and Scallions
    Steamed Broccoli
Beef Tenderloin with Pearl Onions and Mushrooms
    Braised Savoy Cabbage
    Steamed Green Beans
Veal Marsala
    Spaghetti Squash with Garlic and Parmesan
    Green Salad
Grilled Jamaican Jerk Chicken
    Mango Salsa
    Black Beans
Chicken Florentine
    Steamed Asparagus
Chicken Piccata
    Steamed Broccoli and Cauliflower
Mediterranean Couscous with Chicken
    Cucumber and Onion Salad
Curried Apple Chicken Salad Wrap
    Steamed Spinach with Parmesan
    Sliced Red and Yellow Peppers
Pork Tenderloin with Dried Plums and Onions
    Steamed Asparagus
    Spinach or Arugula Salad

Apple Dijon–Encrusted Loin of Pork
   Sugar Snap Peas
   Boiled Baby Red Potatoes
Indian Lamb Stew
   Curried Chickpea and Tomato Salad
Moroccan Spiced Baked Fish
   Casablancan Carrots
   Traditional North African Salad
Citrus Fish Paillard
   Cucumber Slaw
   Sliced Tomatoes
Fish with Fennel, Dill, and Tomatoes
   Waldorf Salad
Zuppa di Pesce (Fish Stew)
   Chopped Endive and Radicchio Salad
   Multigrain Roll
BlueEarth's Thai Basil-Crusted Sea Bass
   Spicy Bok Choy Stir-Fry
Shrimp Creole
   Brown Rice
Vegetarian Lentil Chili
   Green Salad
   Avocado with Lemon
Portobello Parmesan
   Steamed Broccoli Rabe
   Tomato Salad
Goat Cheese and Red Pepper Frittata
   Caesar Salad
   Strawberries with Cool Whip Lite
Summer Squash and Chickpea Stew
   Arugula, White Bean, and Tuna Salad

When you're having dinner guests, or any time you want to prepare something truly special for yourself, browse through this chapter. The meals are arranged as complete menus, so all the planning and coordinating has been done for you. I paired meat and fish dishes with appropriate sides and salads, and calculated exactly what constitutes a serving. I walk you through every step of making a company dinner so you feel confident in the kitchen. Besides making wonderful fare for guests, many of these offerings are special enough to treat family and friends on holidays. The Beef Tenderloin with Pearl Onions and Mushrooms, for example, makes a show-stopping feast at Christmas, and Moroccan Spiced Baked Fish is a perfect entrée to serve at Hanukkah or Rosh Hashanah. If your family has some vegetarians who don't want to eat turkey on Thanksgiving, treat them to Portobello Parmesan (you may find other guests helping themselves to this along with the turkey!).

These luxuriously rich feasts only taste rich. They're calorically controlled so that they are low in fat but high in nutrition and superior in taste. Everyone's enjoying the same menu, yet you're painlessly able to follow your individual 90/10 plan. Once you've planned what you're having as a main course and side dish, check out the fun foods chapter and choose a dessert to go along with it. You'll impress your guests, enjoy a sumptuous meal with them, and not feel bloated and guilty after your dinner party because you've actually stayed with your meal plan.

Menu

Ground Sirloin Steak Smothered in Caramelized Onions
Smashed Yukon Gold Potatoes with Buttermilk and Scallions
Steamed Broccoli

When you're craving good old-fashioned comfort food, this will warm you through and through. Sweet golden caramelized onions top the juicy beef, and the potatoes are creamy and rich.

Ground Sirloin Steak Smothered in Caramelized Onions

Serves 4

1 pound lean ground sirloin
¼ cup chopped red and/or green bell peppers
3 onions, sliced
1 tablespoon vegetable oil
1 teaspoon sugar

1. Mix the beef with the peppers and shape into four oblong patties. Cook *slowly* over medium-low heat for about 20 minutes, or until a meat thermometer registers 170° in the middle.

2. Place the onions and vegetable oil in a nonstick skillet. Cook on high heat for 3 minutes. Reduce the heat to medium-low and continue to cook, stirring frequently, for about 15 minutes. Add sugar to caramelize and cook an additional 5 minutes. Top patties with the onions.

NUTRIENT ANALYSIS

♦ **1 SERVING = 3 OUNCES STEAK**

Calories: 280	Protein: 30 g	Carbohydrates: 6.3 g	Sugar: 2.4 g	Total fat: 15 g
Saturated fat: 4 g	Cholesterol: 64 mg	Sodium: 76.6 mg	Fiber: 1 g	Calcium: 20 mg

Smashed Yukon Gold Potatoes with Buttermilk and Scallions

Serves 6

1 bunch scallions, chopped
1 cup water
¾ cup buttermilk, warmed (not hot)
1¼ pounds Yukon gold potatoes, peeled and cut into 2-inch chunks
Salt and freshly ground black pepper

1. Boil the scallions in 1 cup of water until the water is almost cooked out. Turn off the heat and add the buttermilk.

2. Place the potatoes in a medium saucepan, add enough water to cover, and bring to a boil over high heat. Reduce the heat to moderate and simmer until the potatoes are tender when pierced with a fork, about 30 minutes.

3. Drain the potatoes in a colander and dump them back into the saucepan. With an electric mixer, whip the buttermilk-scallions mixture into the potatoes until thoroughly incorporated. Add salt and pepper to taste.

NUTRIENT ANALYSIS

♦ **1 SERVING = ½ CUP**

Calories: 84	Protein: 3.5 g	Carbohydrates: 17 g	Sugar: 1.7 g	Total fat: 0 g
Saturated fat: 0 g	Cholesterol: 1 mg	Sodium: 36.5 mg	Fiber: 2 g	Calcium: 51.5 mg

1,200-CALORIE PLAN

1 serving steak
1 serving potatoes

1,400-CALORIE PLAN

1 serving steak
1 serving potatoes
1 tablespoon reduced-fat, soft tub margarine
$1/2$ cup steamed broccoli

1,600- & 1,800-CALORIE PLANS

$1^1/_2$ servings steak
1 serving potatoes
$1/2$ cup steamed broccoli

2,000-CALORIE PLAN

$1^1/_2$ servings steak
2 servings potatoes
1 tablespoon reduced-fat, soft tub margarine
$1/2$ cup steamed broccoli

Beef Tenderloin with Pearl Onions and Mushrooms
Braised Savoy Cabbage
Steamed Green Beans

When you want to treat your guests to a truly special meal, try this meltingly tender, very elegant entrée. Pay careful attention to the temperature of the meat during the cooking so that you wind up with rare, medium, or well-done, depending on personal preference.

Beef Tenderloin with Pearl Onions and Mushrooms

Serves 4

1 pound beef tenderloin
Freshly ground black pepper
1 tablespoon olive oil or vegetable oil
1 cup chopped fresh mushrooms
1 cup frozen pearl onions
1 tablespoon minced fresh garlic
Pinch of salt

1. Preheat the oven to 400°.

2. Sprinkle both sides of the beef with pepper. In medium-size nonstick skillet, heat the oil over medium-high heat until hot. Sear and brown the beef on all sides. Set beef aside.

3. In the same hot skillet, sauté the mushrooms and onions until tender. Add the garlic and salt and sauté for an additional minute.

4. Place the beef in an ovenproof pan and cover with mushroom-onion mixture. Roast for 10 to 20 minutes or until the internal temperature reaches 145° for medium rare, or 160° for medium, or 170° for well-done.

◆ **1 SERVING = 3 OUNCE STEAK**

Calories: 234	Protein: 25 g	Carbohydrates: 5 g	Sugar: 2.5 g	Total fat: 12.7 g
Saturated fat: 4 g	Cholesterol: 70 mg	Sodium: 70 mg	Fiber: 1.2 g	Calcium: 51 mg

Braised Savoy Cabbage

Serves 6

2 pounds savoy cabbage, sliced
2 apples, any variety, diced
1 onion, sliced
1 tablespoon vegetable oil
3 tablespoons red wine vinegar
1 tablespoon sugar
1 teaspoon dried thyme

1. Wash the cabbage well and dry thoroughly.

2. In a large nonstick pan, sauté the apples and onion in the oil for 5 minutes, or until the onion is translucent and the apples are slightly caramelized. Add the vinegar, sugar, and cabbage. Cover the pan and cook for 5 to 6 minutes.

3. Add the dried thyme and cook, uncovered, for 2 to 3 minutes.

NUTRIENT ANALYSIS

◆ **1 SERVING = 1 CUP**

Calories: 85	Protein: 3.3 g	Carbohydrates: 20 g	Total Sugar: 9 g	Total fat: 0 g
Saturated fat: 0 g	Cholesterol: 0 mg	Sodium: 43 mg	Fiber: 6 g	Calcium: 62 mg

1,200-CALORIE PLAN

1 serving beef
1 serving cabbage
1 cup steamed green beans

1,400-CALORIE PLAN

1 serving beef
1 serving cabbage
1 cup steamed green beans
1 small whole wheat pita, toasted (no more
   than 70 calories)

1,600- & 1,800-CALORIE PLANS

1½ servings beef
1 serving cabbage
1 cup steamed green beans
1 small whole wheat pita, toasted (no more
   than 70 calories)

2,000-CALORIE PLAN

2 servings beef
1 serving cabbage
1 cup steamed green beans
1 small whole wheat pita, toasted, (no more
   than 70 calories)

Menu

Veal Marsala

Spaghetti Squash with Garlic and Parmesan

Green Salad

Marsala, which is Italy's most famous fortified wine, lends body and richness to this classic veal dish. The garlicky spaghetti squash is easy to make and beautiful to look at. Be sure to pierce the shell of the squash in several places before cooking.

Veal Marsala

Serves 4

¼ cup flour
Salt and freshly ground black pepper
4 four-ounce veal cutlets or scaloppini
3 tablespoons vegetable oil
1 pound mushrooms, sliced
⅔ cup chopped green onions (scallions)
¾ cup low-sodium beef stock
½ cup Marsala wine or sherry
⅓ cup chopped fresh Italian (flat-leaf) parsley

1. Combine the flour, salt, and pepper. Coat the veal slices lightly on both sides with the flour mixture.

2. Add vegetable oil to a skillet. Over medium-high heat, cook the veal for 4 to 5 minutes until golden brown, turning once (veal will not be cooked through). Remove from the pan and set aside.

3. Add the mushrooms and green onions to the skillet and cook for about 5 minutes. Add the beef stock and wine and simmer for about 8 minutes.

4. Return the veal to the skillet and cook until thoroughly heated, about 3 minutes.

5. Serve the veal topped with mushroom sauce. Garnish with chopped fresh Italian parsley.

NUTRIENT ANALYSIS

◆ **1 SERVING = 1 CUTLET**

| Calories: 326 | Protein: 28 g | Carbohydrates: 13 g | Sugar: 4 g | Total fat: 15 g |

| Saturated fat: 2 g | Cholesterol: 89 mg | Sodium: 476 mg | Fiber: 1.6 g | Calcium: 36 mg |

Spaghetti Squash with Garlic and Parmesan

Serves 4

1 spaghetti squash
2 cloves garlic, minced
1 tablespoon olive oil
2–3 tablespoons grated Parmesan cheese

1. Preheat the oven to 350°.

2. Pierce the shell of the spaghetti squash with a fork. Bake, uncovered, for 45 minutes. Turn the squash over and continue to bake until the shell gives to pressure, 15 to 45 minutes, depending on the size.

3. Cut the squash in half and remove and discard the seeds. Remove the spaghettilike strands with a fork.

4. Sauté the garlic in the oil until it's softened but not burned. Add the cooked spaghetti squash strands and toss in the hot pan for 3 minutes.

5. Before serving, sprinkle with Parmesan cheese.

◆ **1 SERVING = ¹/₂ CUP**

| Calories: 74 | Protein: 2 g | Carbohydrates: 5.8 g | Sugar: 0 g | Total fat: 5 g |

| Saturated fat: 1.2 g | Cholesterol: 3 mg | Sodium: 83 mg | Fiber: 0.8 g | Calcium: 72 mg |

1,200-CALORIE PLAN

1 serving veal
Lettuce and cucumbers
2 tablespoons low-calorie dressing

1,400-CALORIE PLAN

1 serving veal
1 serving squash
Lettuce and cucumbers
2 tablespoons low-calorie dressing

1,600- & 1,800-CALORIE PLANS

1¹/₂ servings veal
1 serving squash

2,000-CALORIE PLAN

1¹/₂ servings veal
1 serving squash
Lettuce and cucumbers
2 tablespoons low-calorie dressing
Or
1¹/₂ servings veal
2 servings squash

Menu

Grilled Jamaican Jerk Chicken

Mango Salsa

Black Beans

You'll feel almost like you're in the sunny Caribbean when you sample this classic jerk chicken. The mango salsa offsets it nicely, and the perfect accompaniment is seasoned black beans.

Grilled Jamaican Jerk Chicken

Serves 4

1/2 teaspoon nutmeg
1/2 teaspoon cinnamon
1 tablespoon coriander seeds
1/2 teaspoon allspice
1 teaspoon black peppercorns
1 bunch scallions, chopped
1 large red onion, peeled and quartered
2 to 3 Scotch bonnet peppers or jalapeños
1 teaspoon dried thyme
1 garlic clove
1/4 cup fresh lime juice
1/4 cup sugar
2 pounds boneless, skinless chicken breasts

1. In a blender or food processor pulse everything except the chicken. Pour the mixture over the chicken and marinate in the refrigerator 8 hours or overnight.

2. Grill the chicken on a charcoal fire or bake in a 400° oven until the chicken reaches an internal temperature of 180°.

Note: Reserve 1/4 cup of the marinade for Black Beans (page 198).

◆ 1 SERVING = 1 SIX-OUNCE BREAST

Calories: 286	Protein: 46 g	Carbohydrates: 21 g	Sugar: 14 g	Total fat: 2 g
Saturated fat: 0.6 g	Cholesterol: 103 mg	Sodium: 811 mg	Fiber: 1.8 g	Calcium: 40 mg

Mango Salsa

Serves 4

1 ripe mango, peeled, pitted, and diced
¼ cup diced red bell pepper
⅓ cup coarsely chopped fresh cilantro
2 teaspoons lime juice
1 jalapeño pepper, finely chopped

Toss all ingredients together gently.

◆ 1 SERVING = ⅓ CUP

Calories: 39	Protein: 0.5 g	Carbohydrates: 10 g	Sugar: 7 g	Total fat: 0 g
Saturated fat: 0 g	Cholesterol: 0 mg	Sodium: 4 mg	Fiber: 1.4 mg	Calcium: 10 mg

Black Beans

Serves 4

¼ cup marinade from Grilled Jamaican Jerk Chicken (page 197)
1 can (16 ounces) black beans, drained

In a medium saucepan, bring the marinade and beans to a rolling boil. Cook, stirring, for at least 5 minutes.

◆ 1 SERVING = 1/2 CUP BEANS

Calories: 120	Protein: 7 g	Carbohydrates: 19 g	Sugar: 2 g	Total fat: 1 g

Saturated fat: 0 g	Cholesterol: 0 mg	Sodium: 400 mg	Fiber: 7 g	Calcium: 40 mg

1,200-CALORIE PLAN

1 serving chicken
1 serving salsa
Sliced cucumber

1,600- & 1,800-CALORIE PLANS

1 1/2 servings chicken
1 serving salsa
1/2 cup beans

1,400-CALORIE PLAN

1 serving chicken
1 serving salsa
1/2 cup beans

2,000-CALORIE PLAN

1 1/2 servings chicken
1 serving salsa
3/4 cup beans

Chicken Florentine

Steamed Asparagus

A sumptuous entrée you'd expect to eat in a fine Northern Italian restaurant, this cheese-and-spinach-topped boneless chicken breast is excellent paired with citrus-spritzed steamed fresh asparagus.

Chicken Florentine

Serves 4

¾ cup dry breadcrumbs
¼ cup grated Parmesan cheese
2 large boneless skinless chicken breasts, cut in half
½ cup sliced green onion (scallions)
2 tablespoons olive oil
2 tablespoons flour
1 cup low-sodium chicken stock
1 ten-ounce package frozen chopped spinach, thawed and squeezed dry

1. Preheat the oven to 350°.

2. Mix the breadcrumbs and Parmesan. Dip the chicken breasts in the breadcrumbs and cheese mixture to coat lightly. (Save leftover breadcrumb mixture.) Arrange in a baking dish.

3. In a saucepan, cook the onion in olive oil until tender. Blend in the flour and cook for 1 to 2 minutes. Stir in the chicken stock all at once. Cook, stirring, until thick and bubbly. Stir in the spinach.

4. Spoon the spinach mixture over the chicken and sprinkle with rest of the breadcrumb mixture.

5. Bake, uncovered, for 30 minutes, or until done.

◆ 1 SERVING = 1 BREAST HALF

Calories: 284	Protein: 25 g	Carbohydrates: 24.8 g	Sugar: 1.3 g	Total fat: 10 g
Saturated fat: 2.5 g	Cholesterol: 41 mg	Sodium: 1147 mg	Fiber: 3.7 mg	Calcium: 227 mg

1,200-CALORIE PLAN

1 serving chicken

16 steamed asparagus spears

1,400-CALORIE PLAN

1¹/₂ servings chicken

8 steamed asparagus spears

1,600- & 1,800-CALORIE PLANS

1¹/₂ servings chicken

16 steamed asparagus spears drizzled with
low-fat balsamic vinaigrette

2,000-CALORIE PLAN

2 servings chicken

16 steamed asparagus spears drizzled with
low-fat balsamic vinaigrette

This classic chicken dish has a sauce made from garlic, white wine, and lemon. Be sure to pound the meat extra thin so it cooks quickly.

Chicken Piccata

Serves 4

1½ pounds boneless and skinless chicken breast (about 6 ounces each breast)
½ cup plus 1 teaspoon all-purpose flour
Salt and freshly ground black pepper
¼ cup olive oil
4 cloves garlic, minced
¼ cup lemon juice
½ cup dry white wine
6 tablespoons capers, drained and rinsed
2 tablespoons fresh flat-leaf (Italian) parsley, chopped

1. One at a time, place the chicken breasts between two pieces of waxed paper. Working from the center to the edges, gently pound the chicken with a meat mallet or rolling pin to a thickness of ¼ inch.

2. On a shallow plate, combine ½ cup flour, salt, and pepper. Dip the chicken in the flour mixture to coat all sides.

3. In a saucepan, sauté the olive oil and garlic for 1 minute. Add the chicken and cook until browned but not fully done on both sides. Remove the chicken to a plate and set aside. Add 1 teaspoon of flour to the pan and cook for 1 minute.

4. Add the lemon juice, wine, and capers to the pan and cook over medium heat, scraping the bottom of the pan until it is clean.

5. Return the chicken to the pan for about 8 minutes, until it is cooked through (to 180°) and the sauce has thickened.

NUTRIENT ANALYSIS

♦ 1 SERVING = 1 SIX-OUNCE BREAST

Calories: 350	Protein: 33 g	Carbohydrates: 16.7 g	Sugar: 0.8 g	Total fat: 15 g

Saturated fat: 2 g	Cholesterol: 71 mg	Sodium: 1030 mg	Fiber: 0.6 g	Calcium: 18 mg

1,200-CALORIE PLAN

1 serving chicken
1/2 cup steamed broccoli and cauliflower

1,400-CALORIE PLAN

1 serving chicken
1/2 cup steamed broccoli and cauliflower
1 fist-size baked potato, plain

1,600- & 1,800-CALORIE PLANS

1 1/2 servings chicken
1 cup steamed broccoli and cauliflower

2,000-CALORIE PLAN

1 1/2 servings chicken
1 cup steamed broccoli and cauliflower
1 fist-size baked potato, plain

Mediterranean Couscous with Chicken
Cucumber and Onion Salad

This is Mediterranean comfort food at its best—nutty-flavored couscous, boneless chicken, chickpeas, and other vegetables, all mellowed with cumin and oregano. You can make this dish ahead of time and store in the refrigerator for up to two days. It's good hot or at room temperature.

Mediterranean Couscous with Chicken

Serves 6

2 tablespoons olive oil
12 ounces skinless, boneless chicken breasts,
2 cloves garlic, minced
1 bunch green onions (scallions), trimmed and sliced
2 cups water
1 cup chickpeas (omit for 1,200-calorie plan)
1 sixteen-ounce bag broccoli, cauliflower, and carrots
½ teaspoon cumin
½ teaspoon oregano
1 can (14.5 ounces) salt-free diced tomatoes
1 cup couscous
Salt and freshly ground black pepper

1. In a large, heavy skillet, heat 1 tablespoon olive oil over medium-high heat. Add the chicken and sauté until golden and no longer pink inside. Remove from the skillet, dice the chicken breasts, and set aside.

2. In the same skillet, add the remaining 1 tablespoon olive oil, garlic, and scallions. Sauté for 2 minutes over medium-low heat, being careful not to let the garlic brown.

3. Add the water, chickpeas (remember to omit for 1,200-calorie plan), frozen vegetables, cumin, oregano, and tomatoes to the skillet. Bring to a boil. Stir in the couscous. Cover, remove from the heat, and let stand for 10 minutes.

4. Fluff the mixture with a fork and stir in diced chicken and salt and pepper to taste.

NUTRIENT ANALYSIS

◆ **1 SERVING = 1½ CUPS (ANALYSIS DONE FOR VERSION WITH CHICKPEAS)**

Calories: 320	Protein: 24 g	Carbohydrates: 35 g	Sugar: 3 g	Total fat: 9 g
Saturated fat: 1.8 g	Cholesterol: 47 mg	Sodium: 361 mg	Fiber: 4 g	Calcium: 47 mg

Cucumber and Onion Salad

Serves 6

2 medium cucumbers, very thinly sliced
·1 medium purple onion, thinly sliced
¼ cup white or red vinegar
3 tablespoons sugar
1 tablespoon dried dill

Toss all ingredients and marinate for 1 hour.

NUTRIENT ANALYSIS

◆ **1 SERVING = 1¼ CUPS**

Calories: 45	Protein: 1 g	Carbohydrates: 10.7 g	Sugar: 9 g	Total fat: 0 g	Saturated fat: 0 g
Cholesterol: 0 mg	Sodium: 4 mg	Fiber: 1.2 g	Calcium: 27 mg		

1,200-CALORIE PLAN

1 serving couscous (without chickpeas)

1 serving salad

1,400-CALORIE PLAN

1 serving couscous

1 serving salad

1,600- & 1,800-CALORIE PLANS

1 serving couscous

1 serving salad

1 small whole wheat pita or dinner roll (no
more than 130 calories)

2,000-CALORIE PLAN

1$\frac{1}{2}$ servings couscous

1 serving salad

1 small whole wheat pita or dinner roll
(no more than 130 calories)

Curried Apple Chicken Salad Wrap
Steamed Spinach with Parmesan
Sliced Red and Yellow Peppers

Even people who profess to hate curry like this wrap, in which crunchy apple chunks and pieces of boneless chicken are combined for a light but filling dinner. The steamed spinach and sliced yellow and red peppers lend color to the plate.

Curried Apple Chicken Salad Wrap

Serves 4

2 cups diced, unpeeled tart apples
1 tablespoon lemon juice
1½ pounds cooked chicken breast, diced and chilled
½ cup chopped celery
¼ cup fat-free mayonnaise
¼ cup nonfat plain yogurt
½ cup thinly sliced green onion
2 tablespoons chopped red onion
2 teaspoons curry powder
⅓ cup golden raisins
¾ cup unsalted cashews (omit in 1,200- and 1,400-calorie plans)
4 spinach tortillas (8-inch diameter)

1. In a large bowl, combine the apples and lemon juice. Add the remaining ingredients except tortillas and mix thoroughly.

2. Serve wrapped in the tortillas.

1 SERVING = 1 WRAP (WITHOUT CASHEWS)

| Calories: 350 | Protein: 28 g | Carbohydrates: 52 g | Sugar: 21 g | Total fat: 3.4 g |
| Saturated fat: 1 g | Cholesterol: 59 mg | Sodium: 567 mg | Fiber: 14 g | Calcium: 105 mg |

◆ 1 SERVING = 1 WRAP (WITH CASHEWS)

| Calories: 497 | Protein: 32 g | Carbohydrates: 61 g | Sugar: 22 g | Total fat: 15 g |
| Saturated fat: 3.4 g | Cholesterol: 59 mg | Sodium: 571 mg | Fiber: 14.6 g | Calcium: 116 mg |

1,200-CALORIE PLAN

1 wrap (without cashews)
1/2 cup sliced red and yellow peppers

1,400-CALORIE PLAN

1 wrap (without cashews)
1 cup steamed spinach topped with 1
   tablespoon Parmesan

1,600- & 1,800-CALORIE PLANS

1 wrap (with cashews)
1 cup steamed spinach, plain

2,000-CALORIE PLAN

1 wrap (with cashews)
1 cup steamed spinach topped with 2
   tablespoons Parmesan
Sliced red and yellow peppers

Menu
Pork Tenderloin with Dried Plums and Onions
Steamed Asparagus
Spinach or Arugula Salad

Lean, flavorful boneless tenderloin fillets are succulent and perfectly seasoned in this homey meal. Fresh asparagus lends color and crunch—and plenty of nutrients. Serve with arugula or spinach salad garnished with sliced mushrooms, diced red peppers, red onions, and 1 tablespoon low-fat vinaigrette dressing.

Pork Tenderloin with Dried Plums and Onions

Serves 4

1 tablespoon vegetable oil
4 five-ounce boneless pork tenderloin fillets, fat trimmed
2 cups chopped onions
1 large garlic clove, minced or pressed
2 tablespoons all-purpose flour
1 teaspoon dried thyme
1 cup low-sodium chicken broth or water
½ cup pitted dried plums
3 tablespoons fresh lemon juice
Salt and pepper

1. In a large skillet, heat the oil over medium-high heat. Add the pork and brown on all sides until just cooked through, about 3 minutes per side. Transfer to a plate.

2. Add the onions and garlic to the skillet. Sauté until the onions begin to soften, about 3 minutes. Mix in the flour and thyme. Cook, stirring, for 1 minute. Gradually stir in the broth.

3. Add the plums and lemon juice. Boil, stirring occasionally, until the sauce thickens enough to coat a spoon, about 5 minutes.

4. Return the pork to the skillet. Simmer until heated through, about 2 minutes. Season with salt and pepper to taste.

1,200-CALORIE PLAN

1 serving pork
6 spears steamed asparagus drizzled with
    fresh lemon juice

1,400-CALORIE PLAN

1 serving pork
12 spears steamed asparagus drizzled with
    fresh lemon juice
Spinach or arugula salad

1,600- & 1,800-CALORIE PLANS

1½ servings pork
Spinach or arugula salad

2,000-CALORIE PLAN

1½ servings pork
12 spears steamed asparagus drizzled with
    fresh lemon juice
Spinach or arugula salad

> **Menu**
> Apple Dijon–Encrusted Loin of Pork
> Sugar Snap Peas
> Boiled Baby Red Potatoes
>
> This family-pleasing entrée consists of a loin of pork that's swathed in crunchy breadcrumbs mixed with applesauce before roasting. Sugar snap peas and tiny red potatoes make the meal springlike.

Apple Dijon–Encrusted Loin of Pork

Serves 4

2 tablespoons Dijon mustard
1 teaspoon dried thyme
1 cup plain, unsweetened applesauce
1 pound pork loin
1 cup breadcrumbs

1. Preheat the oven to 325°.

2. Mix the mustard, thyme, and applesauce. Coat the pork loin with the apple mixture, then cover with breadcrumbs, making sure to entirely coat the pork.

3. Place the pork on a rack in a baking pan and roast for 40 minutes, or until the pork reaches an internal temperature of 160°.

NUTRIENT ANALYSIS				
◆ 1 SERVING = 3 OUNCES PORK				
Calories: 310	Protein: 24 g	Carbohydrates: 30 g	Sugar: 9 g	Total fat: 9 g
Saturated fat: 2.5 g	Cholesterol: 48 mg	Sodium: 514 mg	Fiber: 1 g	Calcium: 110 mg

1,200-CALORIE PLAN

1 serving pork
$1/2$ cup steamed sugar snap peas

1,400-CALORIE PLAN

1 serving pork
1 cup steamed sugar snap peas
$1/2$ cup boiled red potatoes, seasoned with
  lemon pepper

1,600- & 1,800-CALORIE PLANS

$1^1/2$ servings pork
$1/2$ cup steamed sugar snap peas
$1/2$ cup boiled red potatoes, seasoned with
  lemon pepper

2,000-CALORIE PLAN

$1^1/2$ servings pork
$1^1/2$ cups steamed sugar snap peas
$1/2$ cup boiled red potatoes, seasoned with
  lemon pepper

This authentic Indian lamb stew prepared with lentils and tomatoes is a good entrée to make on a chilly weekend night when company's coming. The Curried Chickpea and Tomato Salad is an easy-to-make accompaniment.

Indian Lamb Stew

Serves 6

3 tablespoons vegetable oil
1½ cups chopped onion
1 pound lean, trimmed boneless lamb, cut into 1-inch pieces
2 garlic cloves, minced
2 teaspoons minced fresh ginger
3 tablespoons flour
2 cups water
1 can (28 ounces) diced tomatoes in juice
1 cup dried lentils
1 teaspoon ground cumin
½ teaspoon ground coriander
1 ten-ounce package frozen chopped spinach
¼ cup chopped fresh cilantro
About 2 ounces plain nonfat yogurt

1. In a large skillet, heat the vegetable oil. Add the onions and sauté over medium heat for 5 to 7 minutes, until caramelized. Add the lamb, garlic, and ginger. Brown the lamb on all sides, about 4 minutes. Sprinkle in the flour and continue cooking, stirring constantly, for about 2 minutes, until the flour slightly browns.

2. Add the water, tomatoes, lentils, cumin, and coriander. Cook, covered, over medium-low heat for 1 hour, stirring occasionally. Stir in the frozen spinach and cilantro. Cook, uncovered, for 30 minutes.

3. Garnish each serving with 1 teaspoon yogurt.

NUTRIENT ANALYSIS

◆ 1 SERVING = 1¾ CUPS

Calories: 347	Protein: 29 g	Carbohydrates: 32 g	Sugar: 8.4 g	Total fat: 11 g
Saturated fat: 2 g	Cholesterol: 50 mg	Sodium: 561 mg	Fiber: 13 g	Calcium: 182 mg

Curried Chickpea and Tomato Salad

Serves 4

1 ten-ounce can chickpeas, drained and rinsed
1 large ripe tomato, chopped small
6–8 green onions (scallions), sliced
½ cucumber, chopped
Juice of 2 limes
2 tablespoons olive oil
1 teaspoon ground curry (optional)

1. In a medium-size bowl, mix the chickpeas, tomato, onion, and cucumber.

2. In a small bowl, mix the lime juice, olive oil, and curry.

3. Pour the dressing over the salad and toss well.

◆ **1 SERVING = ¾ CUP**

Calories: 116	Protein: 3 g	Carbohydrates: 16 g	Sugar: 1.7 g	Total fat: 5 g
Saturated fat: 0.6 g	Cholesterol: 0 mg	Sodium: 147 mg	Fiber: 3.7	Calcium: 41 mg

1,200-CALORIE PLAN

1 serving stew

1,400-CALORIE PLAN

1 serving stew
1 serving salad

1,600- & 1,800-CALORIE PLANS

1 serving stew
1 serving salad
1 small whole wheat pita (no more than 70 calories), or ½ regular-size pita

2,000-CALORIE PLAN

1½ servings stew
1 serving salad

When you crave something exotic, try this perfectly spiced meal. It's typical of feasts served in North Africa, where spices like coriander and cumin are used to flavor everything from veggies to seafood.

Moroccan Spiced Baked Fish

Serves 6

3 tablespoons olive oil
1 teaspoon ground cumin
1 teaspoons ground coriander
½ teaspoon ground cinnamon
1 clove garlic, finely chopped
Salt and freshly ground black pepper
6 six-ounce fish fillets (cod or flounder)
2 medium onions, sliced
1 diced large tomato or 1 fourteen-ounce can low-salt tomatoes with juice
¼ cup fresh chopped parsley
1 lemon, cut into 6 wedges

1. Preheat the oven to 400°.

2. In a small bowl, mix the oil, spices, garlic, salt, and pepper. Spread the spice mixture on both sides of fish fillets.

3. In the center of a large sheet of aluminum foil lay in half the onions, the fish, and the remaining onions and tomato. Tightly seal the foil, folding over the edges well.

4. Bake for 30 to 40 minutes.

5. Garnish with parsley and serve with a lemon wedge.

Casablancan Carrots

Serves 6

1 pound carrots, peeled and sliced on the diagonal
1 tablespoon sugar
2 tablespoons olive oil
2 tablespoons lemon juice
2 tablespoons cilantro, chopped

1. Boil the carrots for approximately 10 minutes. Drain.

2. Toss with the remaining ingredients.

Traditional North African Salad

Serves 6

3 large green bell peppers, cut in strips
2 medium tomatoes, diced
3 tablespoons olive oil
2 teaspoons lemon juice
2 cloves garlic, minced (optional)
1 teaspoon paprika
Salt
3 cups shredded lettuce

1. Place the peppers in microwave-safe bowl and cover. Cook on high for 5 minutes, until the peppers are tender. Allow to cool.

2. Combine the peppers with the remaining ingredients and mix thoroughly. Cover and refrigerate for 1 hour.

3. Arrange the lettuce on a serving platter and top with the salad.

NUTRIENT ANALYSIS

♦ 1 SERVING = 1 CUP

Calories: 91	Protein: 1.4 g	Carbohydrates: 7.0 g	Sugar: 3.2 g	Total fat: 7.1 g
Saturated fat: 1 g	Cholesterol: 0 mg	Sodium: 7.4 mg	Fiber: 2.1 g	Calcium: 20 mg

♦ **OPTIONAL DESSERT:**

Finish off your meal with big cup of hot mint tea laced with a teaspoon of sugar (or sugar substitute).

1,200-CALORIE PLAN

1 serving fish
1 serving carrots
1 serving salad

1,400-CALORIE PLAN

1 serving fish
1 serving carrots
1 serving salad
1 small toasted whole wheat pita (no more
    than 70 calories)

1,600- & 1,800-CALORIE PLANS

1½ servings fish
1 serving carrots
1 serving salad
1 small toasted whole wheat pita (no more
    than 70 calories)

2,000-CALORIE PLAN

2 servings fish
1 serving carrots
1 serving salad
1 small toasted whole wheat pita (no more
    than 70 calories)

Citrus Fish Paillard
Cucumber Slaw
Sliced Tomatoes

A paillard is a thin piece of meat or fish. In this case, it's seafood, which here is sautéed and lightly spiked with citrus juice. (You can substitute chicken; just make sure to increase the cooking time.) A crisp Cucumber Slaw makes the perfect accompaniment.

Citrus Fish Paillard

Serves 4

4 firm-fleshed fish steaks, about 4 ounces each (marlin, tuna, halibut, or salmon)
3 shallots or 1 medium onion, minced
2 cloves garlic, minced
3 tablespoons olive oil
1 cup white wine
2 tablespoons lemon juice
1 tablespoon lemon zest
1 bunch chopped scallions
Salt and freshly ground black pepper

1. Partially freeze the fish and slice it across the grain about ½-inch thick. Pound with a mallet or rolling pin to an even thickness of about ⅛ inch. Keep the fish refrigerated until ready to use.

2. In a small saucepan, cook the shallots, garlic, and olive oil slowly for 10 minutes. Add the wine and reduce by ¾. Add the lemon juice, lemon zest, scallions, and salt and pepper to taste. Bring to a boil and remove from the heat.

3. Place the fish paillards on heavy-duty aluminum foil. Broil about 4 inches from the heat for 2 minutes. Transfer to warm plates and serve immediately, topped with the sauce.

◆ **1 SERVING = 1 FISH STEAK**

Calories: 285	Protein: 23.5 g	Carbohydrates: 6.3 g	Sugar: 1.8 g	Total fat: 14 g
Saturated fat: 2 g	Cholesterol: 59 mg	Sodium: 84 mg	Fiber: 0.6 mg	Calcium: 43.5 mg

Cucumber Slaw

Serves 4

2 cups shredded unpeeled cucumber, squeezed and patted dry with a paper towel
½ cup shredded peeled carrot
¼ cup fat-free mayonnaise
2 tablespoons Dijon mustard
1 teaspoon dried dill
3 tablespoons lime juice
Salt and pepper

Combine all the ingredients and chill before serving.

◆ **1 SERVING = ABOUT ⅓ CUP**

Calories: 49	Protein: 1.7 g	Carbohydrates: 10.6 g	Sugar: 5.5 g	Total fat: 0 g
Saturated fat: 0 g	Cholesterol: 0 mg	Sodium: 186 mg	Fiber: 1.8 g	Calcium: 41 mg

1,200-CALORIE PLAN

1 serving fish
1 serving slaw

1,400-CALORIE PLAN

1 serving fish
2 servings slaw
Sliced tomatoes
1 tablespoon low-fat vinaigrette dressing

1,600- & 1,800-CALORIE PLANS

1½ servings fish
1 serving slaw
Sliced tomatoes
1 tablespoon low-fat vinaigrette dressing

2000-CALORIE PLAN

2 servings fish
1 serving slaw
Sliced tomatoes, plain

Sweet, delicate fennel is the perfect flavoring for seafood, and the perfect side is Waldorf Salad. It dates back to the 1890s, where it was first served at New York's Waldorf-Astoria Hotel.

Fish with Fennel, Dill, and Tomatoes

Serves 4

1 cup sliced fennel (discard the tough core)
1 cup chopped tomatoes
1 tablespoon fresh lemon juice
4 five-ounce fish fillets
1 teaspoon dried dill

1. Preheat the oven to 500°.

2. Spread the sliced fennel in a baking dish. Cover with the tomatoes and lemon juice, and place the fish on top. Sprinkle with the dill. Cover tightly with aluminum foil.

3. Turn the oven down to 350° and bake the fish for 22 to 25 minutes.

NUTRIENT ANALYSIS

◆ **1 SERVING = 1 FISH FILLET**

Calories: 254	Protein: 15 g	Carbohydrates: 38 g	Sugar: 6.7 g	Total fat: 3.8 g
Saturated fat: 0 g	Cholesterol: 36 mg	Sodium: 599 mg	Fiber: 1.2 g	Calcium: 16 mg

Waldorf Salad

Serves 4

1 tablespoon lemon juice
3 apples, unpeeled, cored, and chopped into bite-size pieces
1 cup seedless red grapes, cut in half
2/3 cup finely chopped celery
1/3 cup fat-free mayonnaise
1/2 cup chopped walnuts (omit for 1,200-calorie plan)
2 cups mixed greens

Sprinkle the lemon juice over apples. Add the grapes, celery, and mayonnaise. Toss. Add the walnuts and toss again. Serve over mixed greens.

NUTRIENT ANALYSIS

◆ **1 SERVING = 1¾ CUPS (ANALYSIS DONE FOR VERSION WITH WALNUTS)**

Calories: 156	Protein: 3 g	Carbohydrates: 29 g	Sugar: 22.8 g	Total fat: 5 g
Saturated fat: 0 g	Cholesterol: 0 mg	Sodium: 183 mg	Fiber: 4.2 g	Calcium: 35 mg

1,200-CALORIE PLAN

1 serving fish
1 serving salad (no walnuts)

1,400-CALORIE PLAN

1 serving fish
1 serving salad

1,600- & 1,800-CALORIE PLANS

1½ servings fish
1 serving salad

2,000-CALORIE PLAN

1½ servings fish
1 serving salad
½ cup cooked basmati rice

Zuppa di Pesce
Chopped Endive and Radicchio Salad
Multigrain Roll

Zuppa di pesce, which means "fish soup" in Italian, is somewhat of a misnomer, as this version is more like a stew. A pungent salad of radicchio and endive contrasts perfectly with the sweetness of the stew.

Zuppa di Pesce (Fish Stew)

Serves 4

1 tablespoon olive oil
1 cup chopped onion
3 garlic cloves, minced
1 celery rib, chopped
2 medium carrots, peeled and cut into disks
2/3 cup chopped fresh Italian flat-leaf parsley
1/4 pound small red potatoes, cut into quarters
1 twenty-eight-ounce can low-salt chopped tomatoes, with juice
1 tablespoon tomato paste
1 tablespoon water plus 1 1/2 cups water
1/2 cup dry white wine
1 teaspoon lemon zest
1 tablespoon fennel seeds
2 pounds white fish of your choice, such as cod, halibut, sole, or bass
Large pinch saffron

1. In a large pot, heat olive oil, then sauté onion, garlic, celery, and carrots for 4 minutes.

2. Add the parsley, potatoes, tomatoes, tomato paste, and 1 tablespoon water and cook for 5 minutes.

3. Add the wine, remaining water, lemon zest, and fennel seeds, and simmer about 20 minutes.

4. Add the fish and saffron, and cook for approximately 20 minutes.

NUTRIENT ANALYSIS

◆ **1 SERVING = 2 CUPS**

Calories: 338	Protein: 44 g	Carbohydrates: 24 g	Sugar: 10 g	Total fat: 5.3 g
Saturated fat: 0.7 g	Cholesterol: 97 mg	Sodium: 407 mg	Fiber: 6.7 g	

1,200-CALORIE PLAN

1 serving stew

1,400-CALORIE PLAN

1 serving stew
1 cup chopped endive and radicchio salad
2 tablespoons low-fat vinaigrette dressing

1,600- & 1,800-CALORIE PLANS

1 serving stew
1 cup chopped endive and radicchio salad
2 tablespoons low-fat vinaigrette dressing
1 small multigrain roll or 1 whole wheat pita, toasted (roll or pita should not exceed 140 calories)

2,000-CALORIE PLAN

1½ servings stew
1 cup chopped endive and radicchio salad
2 tablespoons low-fat vinaigrette dressing
1 small whole wheat pita, toasted (should not exceed 70 calories)

Panko, Japanese breadcrumbs that you can find in Asian markets, are somewhat coarser than our breadcrumbs and yield a perfect, crunchy crust. They're definitely worth searching out for this ginger and basil–perfumed seafood dish.

BlueEarth's Thai Basil-Crusted Sea Bass

Serves 4

4 five-ounce skinless sea bass fillets (not Chilean sea bass)
Salt and freshly ground black pepper
3 tablespoons Thai basil puree (fresh basil leaves ground in a blender)
1 tablespoon ginger juice (grind fresh ginger root and squeeze out the juice)
1 tablespoon Panko crumbs
Olive oil cooking spray

1. Season the sea bass with salt and pepper to taste.

2. In a mixing bowl, combine the basil puree and ginger juice. Rub one side of each fish fillet with the mixture and sprinkle Panko crumbs on the same side.

3. Spray a large saucepan with olive oil cooking spray and heat over a medium flame. Add the fish, crumb side down. Cover and sauté for 3 to 4 minutes.

4. Turn the fish and cook, uncovered, for another 1 to 2 minutes.

◆ **1 SERVING = 1 FISH FILLET**

| Calories: 129 | Protein: 28 g | Carbohydrates: 1 g | Sugar: 0 g | Total fat: 0 g |

| Saturated fat: 0 g | Cholesterol: 0 mg | Sodium: 3 mg | Fiber: 0 g | Calcium: 25 mg |

Spicy Bok Choy Stir-Fry

Serves 4

1 tablespoon light olive oil
1 shallot, sliced
2 tablespoons chopped lemongrass
1 red chili sliced (remove seeds to adjust spice level; fewer seeds = less spicy)
12 ounces yard beans (thin, long green beans) or green beans, trimmed and cut into 1-inch
  pieces
4 pieces baby bok choy, split into 4 pieces each (16 total)
¼ cup vegetable broth
1 cup bean sprouts
1 tablespoon low-sodium soy sauce

1. Heat a wok or large skillet to high. Add oil, shallot, lemongrass, chili, and yard beans. Stir-fry for 2 to 3 minutes.

2. Add the bok choy and broth. Cover and steam the mixture for 1 minute.

3. Add the bean sprouts and soy sauce. Toss together.

◆ **1 SERVING = 1 CUP**

Calories: 76	Protein: 3 g	Carbohydrates: 10 g	Sugar: 2.6 g	Total fat: 3.8 g

Saturated fat: 0.5 g	Cholesterol: 0 mg	Sodium: 211 mg	Fiber: 3.3 g	Calcium: 64 mg

1,200-CALORIE PLAN

1 serving sea bass

2 servings bok choy

Mixed vegetable salad with unlimited lettuce, tomatoes, carrots, onions, peppers, mushrooms, celery, and cucumbers

2 tablespoons low-fat or fat-free salad dressing

1,400-CALORIE PLAN

1 serving sea bass

2 servings bok choy

Mixed vegetable salad with unlimited lettuce, tomatoes, carrots, onions, peppers, mushrooms, celery, and cucumbers

2 tablespoons low-fat or fat-free salad dressing

1/2 cup cooked couscous

1,600- & 1,800-CALORIE PLANS

1 serving sea bass

2 servings bok choy

Mixed vegetable salad with unlimited lettuce, tomatoes, carrots, onions, peppers, mushrooms, celery, and cucumbers

2 tablespoons low-fat or fat-free salad dressing

1 cup cooked couscous

2,000-CALORIE PLAN

2 servings sea bass

2 servings bok choy

Mixed vegetable salad with unlimited lettuce, tomatoes, carrots, onions, peppers, mushrooms, celery, and cucumbers

2 tablespoons low-fat or fat-free salad dressing

3/4 cup cooked couscous

Shrimp Creole

Brown Rice

A full-bodied seafood dish with the flavor of New Orleans, the shrimp is simmered in what chefs call the culinary "holy trinity" of Creole seasonings: chopped green peppers, onions, and celery. Classic Creole cooking combines the flavors of French, Spanish, and African cuisines.

Shrimp Creole

Serves 4

1 tablespoon vegetable oil
1½ cups finely chopped onion
½ cup finely chopped celery
1 clove garlic, pressed or minced
1½ cups finely chopped green pepper
1 can (28 ounces) low-salt diced tomatoes
1 can (28 ounces) low-salt tomato puree
2 tablespoons tomato paste
2 teaspoons Worcestershire sauce
½ teaspoons cayenne
½ teaspoon chili powder
¾ pound medium shrimp, shelled and deveined (1½ pounds shrimp for 1,600/1,800- and 2,000-calorie plans)

1. In a medium skillet, heat the vegetable oil. Add the onion, celery, garlic, and green pepper. Cook until the vegetables are partially tender.

2. Stir in the tomatoes, tomato puree, tomato paste, Worcestershire sauce, cayenne, and chili powder. Bring to full boil, then reduce heat and cook for 5 minutes.

3. Add the shrimp. Bring the mixture to a boil and cook, uncovered, over medium heat for 5 minutes, or until the shrimp are just done.

4. Serve over fluffy brown rice.

NUTRIENT ANALYSIS

♦ 1 SERVING = 2 CUPS

Calories: 291	Protein: 24 g	Carbohydrates: 41 g	Sugar: 19 g	Total fat: 5.5 g
Saturated fat: 0.6 g	Cholesterol: 129 mg	Sodium: 326 mg	Fiber: 10 g	Calcium: 141 mg

1,200-CALORIE PLAN

1 serving shrimp
1 cup spaghetti squash

1,400-CALORIE PLAN

1 serving shrimp
1/2 cup cooked brown rice

1,600- & 1,800-CALORIE PLANS

1 serving shrimp
1 cup cooked brown rice

2,000-CALORIE PLAN

1 1/2 servings shrimp
1 cup cooked brown rice
Or
2 servings shrimp
1 cup spaghetti squash

Vegetarian Lentil Chili

Green Salad

Avocado with Lemon

If you're hosting a meal for vegetarians, this robust, perfectly spiced chili is perfect. Because it's made with lentils in place of dried beans, it's ready in a fraction of the time. A sour cream garnish is a nice touch—be sure to get the fat-free variety. This chili freezes well (but don't add the garnish and sour cream).

Vegetarian Lentil Chili

Serves 6

2 large celery stalks, chopped
1 each green and red bell pepper, chopped in large chunks
1 onion, chopped
½ cup water
4 cloves garlic, minced
2 tablespoons vegetable oil
¾ cup dry lentils
¾ cup dry bulgur wheat
25 ounces low-salt crushed tomatoes (about two 14.5-ounce cans)
6 ounces canned tomato paste
4 cups low-fat, low-sodium vegetable broth
2–4 tablespoons chili powder
1 tablespoon ground cumin
Salt and freshly ground black pepper
Chopped scallions or cilantro, for garnish
Fat-free sour cream, for garnish (see below for amounts per calorie plans)

1. In a large saucepan, combine the celery, peppers, onion, and water. Cook over high heat until the vegetables begin to soften and the water evaporates, about 5 minutes.

2. Add the garlic and vegetable oil, and cook for 3 minutes.

3. Stir in the lentils, bulgur wheat, tomatoes, tomato paste, broth, chili powder, cumin, and salt and pepper to taste. Bring to a boil. Reduce the heat to low and simmer for 30 minutes, or until the lentils are tender.

4. Garnish with scallions or cilantro and sour cream.

NUTRIENT ANALYSIS

♦ **1 SERVING = 1½ CUPS**

Calories: 314	Protein: 15 g	Carbohydrates: 53 g	Sugar: 12 g	Total fat: 7 g
Saturated fat: 0 g	Cholesterol: 0 mg	Sodium: 710 mg	Fiber: 17.4 g	Calcium: 118 mg

1,200-CALORIE PLAN

1 serving chili with 1 tablespoon fat-free sour cream
Green salad with 1 tablespoon low-fat vinaigrette

1,600- & 1,800-CALORIE PLANS

1½ servings chili with 2 tablespoons fat-free sour cream
Green salad with 1 tablespoon low-fat vinaigrette

1,400-CALORIE PLAN

1 serving chili with 1 tablespoon fat-free sour cream
⅓ chopped avocado with lemon juice
Green salad with 1 tablespoon low-fat vinaigrette

2,000-CALORIE PLAN

1½ servings chili with 2 tablespoons fat-free sour cream
⅓ chopped avocado with lemon juice
Green salad with 1–2 tablespoons low-fat vinaigrette

You won't miss the meat in this aromatic hot entrée, in which portobello mushroom caps are stuffed with seasoned breadcrumbs, then blanketed with your favorite low-fat pasta sauce and garnished with fresh basil.

Portobello Parmesan

Serves 4

4 large portobello mushroom caps, cleaned but *not* rinsed
Olive oil cooking spray
Salt and freshly ground black pepper
½ cup seasoned breadcrumbs
2 cups low-fat pasta sauce
½ teaspoon dried oregano
½ teaspoon dried thyme
¼ cup freshly grated Parmesan cheese
2 cups reduced-fat mozzarella cheese
Chopped fresh basil

1. Set the oven to 400°. While the oven is heating, put the mushroom caps, bottom side down, in a shallow baking pan and heat them for 10 minutes. The mushrooms will shrink slightly.

2. Remove the mushrooms from the oven and spray them with the cooking spray. Season with salt and pepper to taste.

3. In an ovenproof baking dish, place the mushrooms bottom side up. Top the mushroom caps with breadcrumbs. Mix the dried herbs with the pasta sauce and cover the mushrooms. Simmer for 4 minutes.

4. Sprinkle the mushrooms with Parmesan and mozzarella. Bake until the cheese melts, about 5 to 10 minutes. Garnish with chopped fresh basil.

NUTRIENT ANALYSIS

◆ **1 SERVING = 1 WHOLE MUSHROOM**

Calories: 272	Protein: 23 g	Carbohydrates: 24 g	Sugar: 2.2 g	Total fat: 9 g
Saturated fat: 6.4 g	Cholesterol: 30 mg	Sodium: 926 mg	Fiber: 3.5 g	Calcium: 546 mg

1,200 CALORIE PLAN

1 mushroom
1 cup broccoli rabe

1,400-CALORIE PLAN

1½ mushrooms
1 cup broccoli rabe

1,600- & 1,800-CALORIE PLANS

1½ mushrooms
1 cup broccoli rabe
1 thickly sliced tomato with vinaigrette
(½ teaspoon olive oil and 2 tablespoons balsamic vinegar)

2,000-CALORIE PLAN

2 mushrooms
1 cup broccoli rabe
1 thickly sliced tomato with 2 tablespoons plain balsamic vinegar

Goat Cheese and Red Pepper Frittata
Caesar Salad
Strawberries with Cool Whip Lite

Tangy goat cheese and sweet red pepper are paired in this savory frittata, which is basically an Italian omelet. It makes a great brunch entrée as well as a satisfying dinner dish, and the fresh berries hint of springtime.

Goat Cheese and Red Pepper Frittata

Serves 2

1 medium onion, chopped fine
1 small red pepper, seeded and diced
1 tablespoon vegetable oil
Salt and pepper, to taste
2–3 cups egg whites or Egg Beaters (2 cups for 1,200-calorie plan; 3 cups for other plans)
2 ounces goat cheese
Fresh basil

1. In a medium-size nonstick skillet, sauté the onion and pepper in oil over medium heat for about 5 minutes. Sprinkle with salt and pepper. Reduce the heat to low.

2. Pour egg whites or Egg Beaters evenly over the vegetable mixture. Stir for the first 3 minutes before the egg begins to set; cook 5 to 7 minutes more, or until the mixture is cooked on the bottom and set on top.

3. Spread the goat cheese over the frittata and cook for an additional 2 minutes until the cheese begins to melt. Sprinkle with fresh basil.

◆ **1 SERVING = ½ RECIPE (USING 2 CUPS EGG WHITES OR EGG BEATERS)**

Calories: 293	Protein: 30 g	Carbohydrates: 13 g	Sugar: 3.4 g	Total fat: 13 g
Saturated fat: 4.6 g	Cholesterol: 13 mg	Sodium: 507 mg	Fiber: 2.1 g	Calcium: 136 mg

◆ **1 SERVING = ½ RECIPE (USING 3 CUPS EGG WHITES OR EGG BEATERS)**

Calories: 353	Protein: 42 g	Carbohydrates: 15 g	Sugar: 4.4 g	Total fat: 13 g
Saturated fat: 4.6 g	Cholesterol: 13 mg	Sodium: 707 mg	Fiber: 2.1 g	Calcium: 176 mg

Caesar Salad

Serves 2

3 cups torn romaine lettuce leaves
2 tablespoons grated Parmesan cheese (for 1,200-calorie plan; 4 tablespoons for other plans)
4 tablespoons fat-free or low-fat Caesar salad dressing (any brand with 30 calories per 2 tablespoons)
¼ cup croutons (for 1,200-calorie plan; ½ cup for other plans)

In a large bowl, toss all the ingredients until thoroughly mixed.

◆ **1 SERVING = 1½ CUPS (ANALYSIS IS FOR ALL PLANS EXCEPT 1,200)**

Calories: 95	Protein: 4.3 g	Carbohydrates: 10.6 g	Sugar: 4.6 g	Total fat: 2.1 g
Saturated fat: 1 g	Cholesterol: 4 mg	Sodium: 1,125 mg	Fiber: 1.8 g	Calcium: 105 mg

1,200-CALORIE PLAN

1 serving frittata (made with 2 cups egg
  whites)
1 serving salad with $1/4$ cup croutons

1,400-CALORIE PLAN

1 serving frittata (made with 3 cups egg
  whites)
1 serving salad with $1/2$ cup croutons

1,600- & 1,800-CALORIE PLANS

1 serving frittata (made with 3 cups egg
  whites)
1 serving salad with $1/2$ cup croutons, and
  extra Parmesan
1 cup sliced strawberries with 2 tablespoons
  Cool Whip Lite

2,000-CALORIE PLAN

$1^{1}/2$ servings frittata (made with 3 cups egg
  whites)
1 serving salad with $1/4$ cup croutons
1 cup sliced strawberries with 1 tablespoon
  Cool Whip Lite

Menu

Summer Squash and Chickpea Stew

Arugula, White Bean, and Tuna Salad

This summery stew is made by simmering zucchini, tomatoes, carrots, and chickpeas. Teamed with Arugula, White Bean, and Tuna Salad, it makes a filling, fiber-rich meal.

Summer Squash and Chickpea Stew

Serves 4

2 tablespoons vegetable oil

1 medium onion, chopped

3 cloves garlic, minced

1 teaspoon oregano

1 teaspoon ground coriander

1 tablespoon flour

2 teaspoons fresh lemon zest

1 can (28 ounces) low-salt chopped tomatoes with juice

1 cup chickpeas, drained and rinsed

2 carrots, halved lengthwise, then thinly sliced

2 cups green and/or yellow zucchini cut in half moons

1 cup vegetable stock

Salt and freshly ground black pepper

1. In a medium-size pan, heat the oil over medium-high heat. Add the onion and cook for about 5 minutes. Add the garlic and cook for additional 1 minute. Add the oregano, coriander, and flour, and cook, stirring for 1 minute. Add the lemon zest, tomatoes, chickpeas, carrots, zucchini, and vegetable stock. Stir well.

2. Cook for 30 minutes, stirring frequently. Season with salt and pepper to taste.

◆ **1 SERVING = 1½ CUPS**

Calories: 204	Protein: 7 g	Carbohydrates: 26.7 g	Sugar: 10.5 g	Total fat: 9 g
Saturated fat: 0 g	Cholesterol: 0 mg	Sodium: 570 mg	Fiber: 7 g	Calcium: 74 mg

Arugula, White Bean, and Tuna Salad

Serves 4

1 can (19 ounces) white cannellini beans, rinsed and drained
1 large rib celery, thinly sliced
½ cup chopped red pepper
2 tablespoons red wine vinegar
1 tablespoon extra-virgin olive oil
1 teaspoon dried dill, oregano, or basil (your choice)
3–4 Roma tomatoes, finely diced
1 large can (12½ ounces) water-packed tuna, drained and flaked (omit in 1,200-calorie plan)
Salt and freshly ground black pepper
1 bunch (4 cups) arugula, washed, stems removed

Place all ingredients except the arugula in a medium bowl. Toss until well combined. Adjust the
seasonings. Serve over the arugula.

NUTRIENT ANALYSIS

◆ **1 SERVING = 2 CUPS (ANALYSIS DONE FOR VERSION WITH TUNA)**

Calories: 248	Protein: 31 g	Carbohydrates: 27 g	Sugar: 3.7 g	Total fat: 5.2 g
Saturated fat: 0.7 g	Cholesterol: 26 mg	Sodium: 788 mg	Fiber: 8.2 g	Calcium: 115 mg

1,200-CALORIE PLAN

1 serving stew
1 serving salad (without tuna)

1,400-CALORIE PLAN

1 serving stew
1 serving salad (with tuna)

1,600- & 1,800-CALORIE PLANS

1 serving stew
1 serving salad (with tuna)
1 small whole wheat pita, toasted (no more than 70 calories)

2,000-CALORIE PLAN

1^1/$_2$ servings stew
1 serving salad (with tuna) and ^{1}/$_2$ cup croutons

Eight

Kids in the Kitchen

Breakfast Pizza
Cheerios French Toast
Egg in a Bread Bed
Peanut Butter and Banana Waffle Sandwich
"Eggs-cellent" Tomato Cheese Omelet
Peanut Butter and Jelly Roll
Whole Wheat Noodles with Spicy Peanut Sauce
Cucumber Tuna Ship
Ham and Cheese Pinwheels
Confetti Chicken Couscous
Frankie and His Friends
Rainbow Chicken Nuggets
Tacos
Banana Choctopus
Chocolate Pudding Sprinkle Cones
Frozen Pudding Lollipops
Fruity Marshmallow Bars
Pretty in Pink Strawberry Soup
Trail Mix

Did you ever look at your child and hope against hope that he or she will grow up not just eating a nutritious diet, but with a healthy attitude toward food? All of us start out in life with the ability to enjoy eating without overdoing it. But sadly, according to the latest research, one-third of American kids are overweight. And by the time many normal weight kids grow up, they too have become overweight and have developed an unhealthy preoccupation with food that manifests itself in many ways. We eat not just to quell hunger pangs, but also when we're bored, busy, sad, angry, or happy—any excuse. Because we grew up hearing from our parents that we couldn't eat dessert until we finished our vegetables, we crave sweets to the point where we gorge ourselves. We're riding the diet roller coaster: bingeing on cookies one day, starving ourselves with lettuce and diet soda the next, then repeating the whole self-defeating cycle.

Obviously, we want our children to grow up with a different attitude. In this chapter, you engage your kids in the kitchen so that they think of cooking as fun and eating as pleasurable. Although children shouldn't diet, the 90/10 eating plan is a healthful strategy for everyone to follow, as it espouses the philosophy that there are no "good" or "bad" foods, no food is off-limits, and there is room in everyone's meal plan for sweets and treats. If you would like your kids to follow along with your personal 90/10 eating plan, that's terrific. Of course, loosen up on the portion control on the 90 percent healthy part, letting your children eat as much as they want, and keep portions for the fun foods the same.

Children take their cues from their parents, so how you eat plays a crucial role in the attitude your children develop toward food. If they see you downing potato chips and then picking at meals because you're full from too much snacking, they'll want to do the same. If they hear you talking about how fat you feel after a dinner pig-out, they'll catch on and echo your words. But if you sit down to a good breakfast in the morning and send positive messages about how food relates to health and energy versus fat and bloat, chances are they will follow suit.

Above all, it's important to give your children ownership of their own food intake. Rather than forcing them to eat a vegetable they despise, provide several options and let them choose. Instead of refusing to let your children eat anything right before dinner because it will "spoil" their appetites, offer them a portion of their meals (or some vegetables) ahead of time to tide them over. Ravenous children are likely to scarf down vegetables like sugar snap peas, baby carrots, or sliced cucumbers and possibly even ask for seconds.

Next, always keep in mind that most kids need to eat more often than grown-ups do. While we're happy with three meals and two snacks, young children seem to eat every couple of hours. That's because they expend so much more energy that they need many more calories than we do. They also tend to eat less at one sitting than most grown-ups. Of course, this doesn't mean they should fill up on sugary doughnuts and Pop Tarts when hunger strikes.

The best way to help kids to choose healthy foods is to practice moderation yourself and encourage them to do the same. You don't need to load up a pizza with every topping in the book, and you don't always have to slather your bagels with cream cheese. Instead, let your child choose one topping (and you choose one) on pizza, and order egg white omelets and oatmeal when your family heads out for breakfast.

By the same token, don't make fast-food restaurants off-limits to your kids. Instead, let them indulge once in a while in a cheeseburger and fries. If you make an issue of it, they'll start to focus more on what they aren't supposed to have and may eventually start bingeing on forbidden treats when they're not with you. In fact, if your kids are fast-food junkies, give them the ownership of this by letting them eat this way one time a week. Let them choose where, when, and what to eat—but make sure they understand that fast-food meals happen only once a week.

Think of cooking with your kids as precious bonding time for both of you. Obviously kitchen supervision is necessary until your children are in their teens. When you cook together, keep repeating to them the basic procedures and safety tips so that you reinforce what they know. Let them work alongside you preparing healthy dishes, and you may be surprised at how much of it they eat.

Your mealtime goal should be to have the whole family enjoying the same healthy, delicious dishes. There is no need to prepare something just for you because you are following the 90/10 plan, because every dish in this book can be enhanced and expanded upon so that the whole family can eat what you make. If you cook healthful foods and eat together as a family now, your children can look forward to a lifetime of feeling good about what they eat and about their appearance.

The kid-friendly meals here range from breakfasts to lunches to fun foods. All are specifically designed for kids—Banana Choctopus, Cucumber Tuna Ship, Frankie and His Friends, Pretty in Pink Strawberry Soup, and more! These meals have been kid-tested and kid-approved: They provide kid-friendly taste and (most of the time) nutrition. They were all created knowing that 90/10 dieters aren't expecting to eat this way. However, the calories are provided for everyone who wants to eat with their children and work the dishes into their own personal meal plan.

Breakfast Pizza

. . . .

Serves 2

If your kids like pizza at any time of day, here's one to brighten their morning. It's quick and easy to make, and you can "customize" it by leaving off the sausage or cheese for anyone in the family who doesn't like these ingredients.

1 whole wheat pita
2 soy sausage links
2 eggs
½ cup shredded low-fat cheese

1. Preheat the oven to 350°.

2. Split and toast the pita.

3. Microwave the sausages according to package directions and cut into thin slices. Set aside.

4. Coat a frying pan with cooking spray and heat over a medium flame. Beat the eggs and scramble them in the pan.

5. Spread the scrambled eggs evenly over both pita halves. Scatter soy sausages over the eggs. Top with shredded cheese.

6. Place the pizzas in the oven until the cheese melts, 1 minute or so.

NUTRIENT ANALYSIS

♦ 1 SERVING = ½ PITA

Calories: 290	Protein: 24 g	Carbohydrates: 23 g	Sugar: 1.3 g	Total fat: 11 g
Saturated fat: 3.7 g	Cholesterol: 222 mg	Sodium: 641 mg	Fiber: 3.4 g	Calcium: 313 mg

Cheerios French Toast

Serves 2

With just a hint of cinnamon, these golden brown slices are delicious served with fresh fruit. And of course, the Cheerios provide fun and pizzazz for your kids. For a lower-calorie/lower-carb version, use 40-calorie wheat bread.

1 small container (8 ounces) egg substitute (or 2 whole eggs and 2 egg whites, beaten)
1 teaspoon ground cinnamon
4 tablespoons skim milk
2 tablespoons sugar (or 1 tablespoon Splenda sugar substitute)
5 heaping tablespoons Cheerios, plain or multigrain
Cooking spray
4 slices whole wheat bread

1. In a medium-size bowl, thoroughly mix the eggs, cinnamon, skim milk, sugar or Splenda, and Cheerios.

2. Spray a large frying pan with cooking spray and heat over a medium-high flame.

3. Dip the bread into the egg-Cheerios mixture, coating both sides. Fry, turning once, until both sides are firm and slightly browned but not burnt.

4. Serve with fresh fruit.

NUTRIENT ANALYSIS

◆ **1 SERVING = 2 SLICES**

Calories: 267	Protein: 18 g	Carbohydrates: 40 g	Sugar: 5 g	Total fat: 2.5 g
Saturated fat: 0 g	*Cholesterol: 1 mg	Sodium: 477.6 mg	Fiber: 5 g	Calcium: 155.5 mg

*Using egg substitute.

Egg in a Bread Bed

Serves 1

Do you remember eating toad-in-the-hole when you were little? This is an updated version of that recipe, and today's kids still love the concept: a hollowed-out slice of bread holds an egg filling. My version is healthier than the ones we used to eat, since it calls for whole wheat rather than white bread and cooking spray instead of butter.

1 slice whole wheat bread
Cooking spray
1 whole egg

1. Cut a circle the size of an Oreo cookie in the middle of the bread.

2. Spray a frying pan with cooking spray and heat over a medium flame. Place the bread in the frying pan. Crack the egg over the bread and allow the yolk to fall into the hole—the white should cover part of the bread and run over into the pan.

3. Cook for 1 minute, then flip and cook for another minute.

NUTRIENT ANALYSIS					
Calories: 144	Protein: 9 g	Carbohydrates: 14 g	Sugar: 1 g	Total fat: 6 g	Saturated fat: 2 g
Cholesterol: 212 mg	Sodium: 212 mg	Fiber: 2 g	Calcium: 45 mg		

Peanut Butter and Banana Waffle Sandwich

Serves 1

Comfort food for kids of all ages, this fun sandwich is good at any time of day. Make sure your banana's nice and ripe so the filling will be sweet and soft, as it should be.

2 frozen whole-grain waffles (preferably calcium fortified)
1 banana
2 tablespoons peanut butter
Carrot sticks, for garnish

1. Toast both waffles and spread a thin layer of peanut butter on each.

2. Peel the banana and slice it into ¼-inch circles.

3. Arrange the banana slices evenly on top of the peanut butter on one waffle. Top with the remaining waffle. Cut into quarters. Garnish with carrot sticks.

NUTRIENT ANALYSIS

Calories: 438	Protein: 14 g	Carbohydrates: 71 g	Sugar: 25 g	Total fat: 15 g
Saturated fat: 3 g	Cholesterol: 0 mg	Sodium: 681 mg	Fiber: 7.8 g	Calcium: 317 mg

"Eggs-cellent" Tomato Cheese Omelet

Serves 1

A great way to pack protein and calcium into your child's morning! Even kids who hate eggs may like this omelet, thanks to a savory filling of melted cheese and chopped fresh tomatoes.

Cooking spray
1 whole egg

2 egg whites
2 tablespoons chopped tomatoes
2 slices low-fat or fat-free cheese
Salt

1. Coat a frying pan with cooking spray. Heat over a medium flame.

2. Beat the egg with the egg whites and pour into the heated pan. When the bottom of the eggs begins to settle, carefully flip onto the other side. Add the tomatoes evenly throughout, and place the cheese on only one side.

3. Fold over the noncheese half to create an omelet. Gently press with a spatula. Lightly sprinkle salt over the omelet.

NUTRIENT ANALYSIS

Calories: 174   Protein: 21.5 g   Carbohydrates: 8.6 g   Sugar: 4.8 g   Total fat: 5 g

Saturated fat: 1.6 g   Cholesterol: 217.5 mg   Sodium: 812 mg   Fiber: 0.3 g

Calcium: 337.9 mg

Peanut Butter and Jelly Roll

Serves 1

Kid-friendly "sushi"! A classic roll-up that's excellent for a school lunchbox or picnic fare, this is a sweet spiral sandwich that's fun for kids to make. Use whatever flavor of jelly or jam they like, so long as it's low in sugar.

2 slices whole wheat bread
2 tablespoons peanut butter
2 tablespoons jelly or jam (preferably low-sugar or sugar-free)

1. With a rolling pin or large soup can, completely flatten out both slices of bread. Cut off the crusts.

2. Spread 1 tablespoon peanut butter on each slice of bread. Top with 1 tablespoon jelly.

3. Roll each slice into a tight spiral. Cut each spiral into 4 slices.

Whole Wheat Noodles with Spicy Peanut Sauce

Serves 4

I often refer to this yummy dish as "peanut butter spaghetti." It's an Asian-flavored entrée studded with fresh veggies and spiked with soy sauce and rice wine vinegar. It's a great make-ahead dish to take to a picnic, and it's just as good cold as at room temperature.

12 ounces whole wheat spaghetti
1 tablespoon sesame oil
¼ cup peanut butter
¼ cup chicken broth
¼ cup low-sodium soy sauce
1 tablespoon sugar
1 tablespoon rice wine vinegar
½ teaspoon hot sauce or Tabasco sauce
Salt and freshly ground black pepper
1 small cucumber, peeled, seeded, and chopped
6 baby carrots, chopped (about ½ cup)
½ cup minced scallions

1. In a large pot of boiling, salted water, cook the whole wheat spaghetti according to package directions, until al dente. Drain the spaghetti, rinse in cold water, and toss with the sesame oil.

2. In a small bowl, combine the peanut butter, broth, soy sauce, sugar, vinegar, and hot sauce. Stir until smooth. Add salt and pepper to taste, and a little extra hot sauce if you like.

3. Toss the noodles with the sauce. Add the chopped cucumber, carrots, and half the scallions. Toss to combine. Spoon into a serving bowl and top with the remaining scallions. Serve cold or at room temperature.

NUTRIENT ANALYSIS

◆ **1 SERVING = 1½ CUPS**

Calories: 468	Protein: 18.9 g	Carbohydrates: 78.5 g	Sugar: 8.6 g	Total fat: 10.9 g
Saturated fat: 1.7 g	Cholesterol: 1.6 mg	Sodium: 729.4 mg	Fiber: 8.8 g	Calcium: 54.9 mg

Cucumber Tuna Ship

Serves 2

If you're, umm, fishing around for a new way to serve your kids tuna, try this eye-catching, veggie-rich salad. They'll love the cucumber "ship," carrot stick "sailing masts," and satisfying, crunchy filling.

1 cucumber, peeled
1 six-ounce can water-packed tuna
1 tablespoon low-fat mayonnaise
Optional for tuna salad: chopped celery, minced onion, and ½ teaspoon mustard
2 baby carrots

1. Hollow out the peeled cucumber.

2. Drain and mash the tuna. Mix with the mayonnaise. You can add celery, minced onion, and mustard. Stuff the tuna salad into the hollowed-out cucumber.

3. Slice the baby carrots in half lengthwise. Place the 4 carrot sticks into the tuna salad to look like sailing masts.

4. Cut the cucumber into two thick pieces (ships).

NUTRIENT ANALYSIS

◆ **1 SERVING = 1 SHIP**

Calories: 156	Protein: 22 g	Carbohydrates: 8 g	Sugar: 5.4 g	Total fat: 3.9 g
Saturated fat: 0 g	Cholesterol: 38 mg	Sodium: 424 mg	Fiber: 2 g	Calcium: 48.3 mg

Ham and Cheese Pinwheels

Serves 1

Even a preschooler can help make this easy roll-up, which makes a great lunch for kids who like their food to be nice and plain. Those who want to spice things up a little can spread some deli-style mustard on the tortilla before layering on the ham and cheese.

1 whole wheat tortilla
2 ounces ham, sliced
1 ounce low-fat American cheese, sliced

1. Evenly lay out the sliced ham on the tortilla. Layer with the sliced cheese.

2. Roll the tortilla into a tight spiral. Slice into quarters.

NUTRIENT ANALYSIS

◆ **1 SERVING = 1 PINWHEEL**

Calories: 215	Protein: 22.6 g	Carbohydrates: 31.6 g	Sugar: 3 g	Total fat: 3.7 g
Saturated fat: 1 g	Cholesterol: 26.6 mg	Sodium: 578 mg	Fiber: 2.6 g	Calcium 227.8 mg

Confetti Chicken Couscous

Serves 6

Colorful, crunchy, and just slightly exotic, this one-dish meal's got all the flavors kids like: raisins, carrots, peas, and chicken. How much curry powder to stir in depends on how spicy your kids like their food.

¾ pound boneless, skinless chicken breast, pounded thin
Salt
½ teaspoon garlic powder
4 large carrots, peeled and diced
¾ cup frozen peas
2 small zucchini, ends removed, diced
½ red bell pepper, cored, seeded, and diced
1½ cups chicken broth (preferably low-sodium)
¼ teaspoon cinnamon
½ teaspoon curry powder
1½ cups instant couscous
3 tablespoons raisins (optional)

1. Heat a stovetop grill or frying pan over medium-high heat. Place the chicken on the grill and sprinkle with salt and garlic powder. Grill 3 minutes, then turn and grill on the other side. When the chicken is done, remove and set aside to cool.

2. In a large pot of boiling, salted water, cook the carrots for 2 minutes. Add the peas and cook for 1 minute. Add the zucchini and red pepper and cook another minute. Remove and drain.

3. Dice the grilled chicken into bite-sized pieces.

4. In a saucepan, bring the chicken broth to a boil. Add the cinnamon and curry powder. Stir in the couscous. Cover the pan, remove it from the heat, and allow to stand for 5 minutes. Fluff the couscous with a fork.

5. Place the couscous in a large serving bowl. Add the vegetables, diced chicken, and raisins. Toss to combine.

- **1 SERVING = 1½ CUPS**

Calories: 348	Protein: 23.3 g	Carbohydrates: 48.3 g	Sugar: 5.7 g	Total fat: 6.8 g
Saturated fat: 1.7 g	Cholesterol: 69.2 mg	Sodium: 134.3 mg	Fiber: 4.9 g	Calcium: 38 mg

Frankie and His Friends

Serves 3

This meal will certainly make your kids laugh—and you too! Fun to look at as well as to eat, this consists of a hot dog "man" standing atop fiber-rich beans. Best of all, it's fast, since both the franks and the beans can be cooked in the microwave.

3 fat-free or low-fat hot dogs
1 sixteen-ounce can vegetarian baked beans
Mustard

1. Boil or microwave the hot dogs.

2. Cook the baked beans on the stove or in the microwave. Place the cooked baked beans in 3 bowls.

3. Take a hot dog and cut from center down to create 2 legs.

4. On the top half of the hot dog, cut slits on either side to create arms.

5. Place one hot dog in each bowl of beans (standing or leaning).

6. Using mustard, create 2 eyes, nose, and mouth.

- ◆ **1 SERVING = 1 HOT DOG WITH ⅓ OF BEANS**

Calories: 179	Protein: 13.4 g	Carbohydrates: 33.4 g	Sugar: 9.6 g	Total fat: 0 g
Saturated fat: 0 g	Cholesterol: 15 mg	Sodium: 980 mg	Fiber: 7.7 g	Calcium: 79.6 mg

Rainbow Chicken Nuggets

Serves 4

The crunchy, colorful coating on these tender nuggets makes them anything but boring—and kids love the slightly sweet taste the crushed cereal imparts. If you don't mind a mess, let your kids crush the cereal. If you prepare them early in the day and refrigerate them unbaked, you'll need to extend the baking time by about 5 minutes.

1 pound boneless, skinless chicken breast
2 egg whites
2 cups Fruity Pebbles cereal, slightly crushed
1 cup fresh breadcrumbs
Cooking spray

1. Preheat the oven to 350°.

2. Pound the chicken to ½-inch thickness. Trim away any visible fat. Cut into about 8 pieces.

3. In a shallow bowl, lightly beat the egg whites with a fork.

4. On a plate, mix the Fruity Pebbles and breadcrumbs.

5. Dip the chicken pieces into the egg white. Then roll them in the Fruity Pebbles mixture to thoroughly coat on all sides.

6. Lightly spray a baking pan with cooking spray. Arrange the chicken in a single layer in the baking pan. Bake for 15 minutes, or until the chicken is thoroughly cooked.

◆ **1 SERVING = 2 NUGGETS**

Calories: 360	Protein: 26 g	Carbohydrates: 38 g	Sugar: 9 g	Total fat: 11 g

Saturated fat: 2.8 g	Cholesterol: 94.4 mg	Sodium: 414.4 mg	Fiber: 0.6 g	Calcium: 71.4 mg

Tacos

Serves 7

You might want to plan a taco party on the night you prepare this recipe—they're great for sleepovers and din-ner play dates. Arrange the taco shells, meat filling, cheese, tomato, and lettuce in separate bowls, assembly line style, and let everyone customize his or her own.

1 pound extra-lean ground turkey breast
Taco sauce flavor packet, mild or hot (1½ ounces)*
1 large red tomato, finely chopped
2 cups chopped or shredded lettuce
1 cup shredded low-fat cheddar cheese
7 hard taco shells

*If your children don't like spicy food, skip the taco sauce and instead stir in ¼ cup marinara sauce. You can further season with pepper and garlic.

1. In a skillet, brown the turkey. Drain off the fat.

2. In a saucepan, mix the seasoning packet and water. Bring to a boil, then lower the heat and simmer, stirring occasionally, for 5 to 6 minutes.

3. In 3 separate bowls, arrange the lettuce, tomato, and cheese.

4. Spoon the turkey meat into the taco shells. Let children garnish their taco shells with tomato, lettuce, and cheese.

Banana Choctopus

Serves 1

One chocolate head and eight banana legs equal one fun-to-eat octopus that kids can help to make. For best results, use a banana that is still slightly firm.

1 banana
Light chocolate syrup

1. Peel the banana and slice it in half. Then slice each half lengthwise into four strips.

2. Squirt about 1 tablespoon chocolate syrup into the middle of a plate—this is the octopus head.

3. Arrange the 8 banana strips around the head as the octopus legs.

NUTRIENT ANALYSIS

Calories: 149	Protein: 1.6 g	Carbohydrates: 38.7 g	Sugar: 20 g	Total fat: 0.7 g
Saturated fat: 0.3 g	Cholesterol: 0 mg	Sodium: 19.1 mg	Fiber: 3.2 g	Calcium: 9.7 mg

Chocolate Pudding Sprinkle Cones

Serves 6

Instead of ice cream, these colorful cones hold creamy chocolate pudding that's topped with rainbow sprinkles for an extra-festive touch. A good party treat since it's finger food, these are best made slightly ahead of time and refrigerated for 1–2 hours before serving. Do not let the cones sit too much longer in the fridge or they'll become soggy.

1 package (3.9 ounces) Jell-O instant chocolate pudding mix
2 cups skim milk, cold
6 flat-bottom wafer ice cream cones, multicolor pack (green, pink, and basic beige)
Colored sprinkles

1. In a large bowl, prepare the chocolate pudding according to package directions using skim milk.

2. Pour the chocolate pudding evenly into 6 flat-bottom cones.

3. Sprinkle 1 teaspoon multicolored sprinkles on top of each pudding cone.

4. Refrigerate for at least 1 hour. Be sure to set the pudding cones on a stable tray that is out of the way from being knocked over or in a container that keeps them from falling over on their sides.

NUTRIENT ANALYSIS

◆ **1 SERVING = 1 CONE**

Calories: 105	Protein: 4 g	Carbohydrates: 18.8 g	Sugar: 7 g	Total fat: 1.4 g
Saturated fat: 1 g	Cholesterol: 1.5 mg	Sodium: 126.1 mg	Fiber: 0.3 g	Calcium: 107.3 mg

Frozen Pudding Lollipops

Serves 10

Better than ordinary lollipops (fewer than 6 grams of sugar), these rich confections have a surprise layer of chocolate syrup and colored sprinkles. Make them at least 4 hours before you plan to serve them so they have time to freeze. If you like, assemble them a day or two ahead and store them, well wrapped, in the freezer.

1 package instant chocolate pudding mix, fat-free and sugar-free
2½ cups skim milk
2 tablespoons light chocolate syrup
½ cup colored sprinkles or small candies
10 small paper cups
10 wooden Popsicle sticks

1. In a large bowl, blend the pudding mix, milk, and chocolate syrup until thickened and thoroughly mixed.

2. Place 10 paper cups on a baking sheet and spoon 1 teaspoon of sprinkles or candies into the bottom of each. Pour pudding mixture evenly into each cup. Cover with tin foil.

3. Make small holes in the foil and insert a wooden stick into each pudding-filled cup.

4. Place the baking sheet in freezer for 4+ hours (or until the pudding pops are frozen). Remove the foil and tear away the paper cups.

NUTRIENT ANALYSIS

◆ **1 SERVING = 1 POP**

Calories: 90	Protein: 2.9 g	Carbohydrates: 13.7 g	Sugar: 5 g	Total fat: 3 g
Saturated fat: 2.5 g	Cholesterol: 0 mg	Sodium: 72 mg	Fiber: 0 g	Calcium: 85 mg

Fruity Marshmallow Bars

Makes 2 dozen

Reminiscent of that old standby, Rice Krispies treats, these rainbow-colored cookies are big and satisfying to anyone with a serious tooth. Okay, I admit, there's not much nutrition. On the other hand, it's a fun treat for fewer than 100 calories and 1 gram of fat. Be sure to add the cereal when the marshmallow mixture is still hot, so that it's easy to stir.

1 large bag (10½ ounces) miniature marshmallows
2 tablespoons reduced-fat, soft tub margarine
6 cups Fruity Pebbles cereal (or multi-colored Rice Krispies)
Cooking spray

1. In a large glass mixing bowl, combine the marshmallows and margarine. Microwave on high for 1 minute. Remove and stir. Microwave for another 20 seconds, or until gooey and melted. Stir well.

2. Add the Fruity Pebbles (or Rice Krispies) and stir until they are well coated with marshmallow mixture.

3. Spray a glass 9" × 13" baking pan with cooking spray. Spoon and scrape the marshmallow-cereal mixture into the pan. Moisten your fingers with cold water, then press the mixture firmly with your fingers to spread it evenly in the pan. When thoroughly cool, cut into 24 bars.

NUTRIENT ANALYSIS				
◆ 1 SERVING = 1 BAR				
Calories: 82	Protein: 0 g	Carbohydrates: 18.3 g	Sugar: 11 g	Total fat: 0.8 g
Saturated fat: 0 g	Cholesterol: 0 mg	Sodium: 73 mg	Fiber: 0 g	Calcium: 0 mg

Pretty in Pink Strawberry Soup

Serves 6

This cool and creamy soup makes a refreshing dessert, though it tastes pretty good for breakfast, too. You can make the soup several hours before serving time and store it, tightly covered, in the refrigerator.

1 twelve-ounce bag frozen whole strawberries (no sugar added), thawed
5 tablespoons Splenda
1 twelve-ounce can fat-free evaporated milk
1½ cups apple juice or cider
2 tablespoons honey
Juice of ½ lemon
Fat-free whipped cream, for garnish

1. In mixing bowl, stir together the strawberries and the Splenda. Puree it in a food processor or with a hand mixer until smooth.

2. Add the milk, apple juice, honey, and lemon juice. Puree just until smooth.

3. Pour the soup into large bowl and chill for 2 or 3 hours.

4. Ladle the soup into bowls. Garnish each with a dollop of whipped cream.

NUTRIENT ANALYSIS

◆ **1 SERVING = 1 CUP**

Calories: 155	Protein: 4.9 g	Carbohydrates: 34 g	Sugar: 20 g	Total fat: 1.1 g
Saturated fat: 0.6 g	Cholesterol: 4.9 mg	Sodium: 74 mg	Fiber: 1.6 g	Calcium: 209.4 mg

Trail Mix

Serves as many kids as you'd like

This is a great snack and project for younger kids (ages two to six). Not only do they feel proud about preparing their own snack, but they also get the chance to practice their math skills and shake their stuff!

½–1 cup Multi-Grain Cheerios
½–1 cup minipretzels (preferably oat bran)
½ cup raisins
½–1 cup Goldfish crackers
½ cup milk chocolate chips
½–1 cup peanuts

1. Give each child a snack-size ziplock plastic bag.

2. Have each child count out 10 Cheerios and place into the bag.

3. Have each child count out 9 pretzels and place into the bag.

4. Have each child count out 8 raisins and place into the bag.

5. Have each child count out 7 Goldfish crackers and place into the bag.

6. Have each child count out 6 chocolate chips and place into the bag.

7. Have each child count out 5 peanuts and place into the bag.

8. Tightly close the plastic bags and have all children stand up and do the twist. The kids will have fun shaking up the contents of their trail mix. It's also a great idea to put on the song "Twist and Shout" while the kids have fun twisting around.

◆ **1 SERVING = 1 BAG: 10 CHEERIOS, 9 MINIPRETZELS, 8 RAISINS, 7 GOLDFISH, 6 CHOCOLATE CHIPS, 5 PEANUTS**

Calories: 105 | Protein: 2.8 g | Carbohydrates: 14.5 g | Sugar: 5 g | Total fat: 4.6 g

Saturated fat: 1 g | Cholesterol: 1.3 mg | Sodium: 149.6 mg | Fiber: 1.1 g | Calcium: 17.4 mg

Nine

90/10 *Fun Food* Favorites!

Angel Food Cake with Fresh Berries
Lemon Ginger Pudding Cake
Strawberry-Topped Cheesecake
Chocolate Banana Bread
Chunky Applesauce Pie
Creamy Pumpkin Pie
Ice Cream Berry Pie
Oreo Vanilla Pudding Pie
Peanut Butter Pie
Chocolate Chip Meringues
Fudgy Brownie Squares
Ice Cream Cookie Sandwiches
Rebecca's Oatmeal Chip Cookies
Stovetop S'mores
Chocolate Mousse
Microwave Chocolate Pudding
BlueEarth's Pineapple Lemongrass Skewers
Frosty Apple Smoothie
Cranberry Couscous
Oven-Baked French Fries
Garlic Smashed Potatoes
Guacamole
Hot Artichoke Dip

Here are recipes for snacks, sweets, dinner starches, and treats—all delicious dishes you can rely on to satisfy you when you feel the urge to splurge. And you know the drill: 250 calories or fewer per serving. When you want to make a showy dessert for family or company, when you need a savory munchie to serve at a gathering, or when you want to prepare something special for yourself, this is the chapter to turn to. All the items are portion controlled, from Fudgy Brownie Squares to decadent low-fat Peanut Butter Pie. I allotted generous portions, too, which means that you can enjoy 2 small brownies, 6 Chocolate Chip Meringues, or a full ¾ cup of Cranberry Couscous as one serving. And while most foods hit my 250-calorie fun food allotment, others don't even come close. That's because foods like Garlic Smashed Potatoes and low-sugar, low-fat Chocolate Mousse are less caloric for an appropriate portion size. If you do the math and increase the amounts, that's fine. However, I strongly encourage you to stick with the listed portions. Learning to practice portion-controlled eating is the primary key to successful weight management.

Angel Food Cake with Fresh Berries

Serves 8

A heavenly way to show off ripe strawberries, this tall, pure white cake is light and fluffy. If you like, substitute fresh raspberries for the strawberries, or mix equal parts of strawberries, raspberries, and blueberries.

1 cup cake flour
1½ cups granulated sugar
14 egg whites
1½ teaspoons cream of tartar
1½ teaspoons vanilla extract
½ teaspoon lemon extract
¼ teaspoon salt
¼ cup confectioner's sugar
2 cups fresh strawberries, sliced

1. Preheat the oven to 375°.

2. Sift together the flour and ¾ cup sugar.

3. Place the egg whites into the work bowl of an electric mixer. Whip on low speed just until foamy. Add the cream of tartar, vanilla extract, lemon extract, and salt. Beat at high speed until soft peaks form. Gradually add the remaining ¾ cup sugar. Beat until the peaks are stiff but not dry.

4. Sift the flour into the beaten egg whites in three batches, beating on low speed just until mixed.

5. Scrape the batter into a 10-inch tube pan, preferably with a removable bottom, smoothing out the top. Run a knife through the batter a few times to get rid of air bubbles.

6. Bake the cake in the lower third of the oven for 30 to 40 minutes, until the top springs back when you press on it with your finger.

7. Invert the cake pan onto the neck of a bottle. Allow it to cool in the pan for several hours. Then run a knife around the edges of the cake to loosen it, and ease the cake onto a serving plate. If your pan has a removable bottom, you can just lift out the cake.

8. Dust the top of the cake with confectioner's sugar. Cut the cake with a serrated knife. Serve each slice with ¼ cup sliced fresh strawberries.

NUTRIENT ANALYSIS

◆ **1 SERVING = 1 SLICE (⅛ OF CAKE) WITH ¼ CUP BERRIES**

Calories: 245 | Protein: 7.5 g | Carbohydrates: 53 g | Sugar: 40 g | Total fat: 0 g

Saturated fat: 0 g | Cholesterol: 0 mg | Sodium: 170 mg | Fiber: 1 g | Calcium: 11 mg

Vitamin C: 20 mg

Lemon Ginger Pudding Cake

Serves 6

One of my favorite desserts, this offers a nice contrast between cake and dense pudding—with an intense lemon flavor. The cake is best served at room temperature or slightly warm.

3 eggs, separated
½ cup skim milk
¼ cup freshly squeezed lemon juice
1½ teaspoons freshly grated lemon peel
½ teaspoon ground ginger
¼ cup sugar
¼ cup Splenda
⅓ cup flour
Pinch of salt
Vegetable oil spray
Lemon slices, for garnish

1. Preheat the oven to 350°.

2. In a mixing bowl, beat the egg yolks only. Add the skim milk, lemon juice, lemon peel, and ginger. Beat well. Add the sugar, Splenda, flour, and salt. Beat until smooth.

3. In a separate bowl, beat the egg whites until stiff peaks form. Gently fold the yolk mixture into the beaten egg whites.

4. Pour the entire mixture into a loaf pan sprayed with cooking spray. Place the baking pan in a larger pan and pour water into the pan to a depth of 1 inch. Bake for 25 to 30 minutes, until golden.

5. Allow the cake to cool slightly. Cut into 6 slices. Arrange thin slices of fresh lemon around the cake for a decorative look.

NUTRIENT ANALYSIS

◆ **1 SERVING = 1 SLICE (⅙ OF CAKE)**

Calories: 105	Protein: 4.5 g	Carbohydrates: 16 g	Sugar: 9 g	Total fat: 2.6 g
Saturated fat: 1 g	Cholesterol: 106 mg	Sodium: 237 mg	Fiber: 0 g	Calcium: 60 mg

Strawberry-Topped Cheesecake

Serves 8

This classic cream cheese confection in a graham cracker crust features a topping of fresh strawberries. For the easiest preparation, allow the cream cheese to soften for at least 1 hour before you plan to prepare the filling. Be sure to refrigerate leftovers.

CRUST
1 cup low-fat graham cracker crumbs
2 tablespoons Splenda
¼ cup reduced-fat, soft tub margarine, melted

FILLING
12 ounces (4 three-ounce packages) fat-free cream cheese, softened
1 egg
1 egg white

½ cup sugar
¼ cup Splenda
¾ teaspoon vanilla extract
2 teaspoons freshly grated lemon peel

TOPPING
1 cup sliced fresh strawberries

1. Preheat the oven to 350°.

2. Make the crust: In a small mixing bowl, combine the crumbs, Splenda, and margarine. Use the back of a metal spoon to press the crust onto the bottom and sides of an 8-inch pie pan.

3. Make the filling: In a medium mixing bowl, with the electric mixer set on medium speed, beat the cream cheese, egg, egg white, sugar, Splenda, vanilla extract, and grated lemon peel.

4. Spoon and scrape the filling into the prepared pie shell. Bake the pie for 40 to 45 minutes, until the filling is set.

5. Chill well. Top with sliced fresh strawberries.

NUTRIENT ANALYSIS				
◆ 1 SERVING = 1 SLICE (⅛ OF PIE)				
Calories: 150	Protein: 7 g	Carbohydrates: 22 g	Sugar: 14 g	Total fat: 4 g
Saturated fat: 1 g	Cholesterol: 30 mg	Sodium: 383 mg	Fiber: 1.3 g	Calcium: 58 mg

Chocolate Banana Bread

Serves 8

Two favorites we never outgrow—chocolate and bananas—team up in this delicious bread that's as satisfying as cake. The riper the bananas, the sweeter the bread will be. You can freeze this loaf, well wrapped, for up to three months.

½ cup reduced-fat, soft tub margarine
¾ cup Splenda
2 eggs, beaten
2 mashed bananas
¼ cup skim milk
1 teaspoon vanilla extract
2 cups all-purpose flour
¼ cup baking cocoa
1 teaspoon baking soda
1 teaspoon salt
Cooking spray

1. Preheat the oven to 350°.

2. In a mixing bowl, cream together the margarine, Splenda, eggs, bananas, milk, and vanilla.

3. In a separate bowl, mix the flour, cocoa, baking soda, and salt.

4. Combine both mixtures.

5. Spray a loaf pan with cooking spray and pour in the batter. Bake for 1 to 1¼ hours, or until an inserted toothpick comes out clean. Slice into 8 equal servings.

◆ **1 SERVING = 1 SLICE (⅛ LOAF)**

Calories: 228	Protein: 5.6 g	Carbohydrates: 35 g	Sugar: 6 g	Total fat: 7.3 g

Saturated fat: 1.5 g	Cholesterol: 53 mg	Sodium: 552 mg	Fiber: 1.5 mg	Calcium: 77 mg

Chunky Applesauce Pie

Serves 6

Homemade applesauce lightly spiced with cinnamon fills store-bought "mini" graham cracker piecrusts in a homey dessert that's especially satisfying in the fall. To keep the crusts nice and crisp, fill them as close as possible to serving time. (An apple corer/slicer gadget makes the job easier.)

5 medium apples (a mixture of whatever types are in your grocery)
⅓ cup water
¼ teaspoon vanilla extract
¼ teaspoon ground cinnamon
⅛ teaspoon nutmeg
6 Keebler "mini" graham cracker piecrusts (120 calories each)

1. Core and cut the apples into 8 wedges each.

2. In a large saucepan, combine the apples, water, vanilla, cinnamon, and nutmeg. Simmer covered, for 15+ minutes, or until apples are part sauce with some chunks of apple left. Watch closely and stir often to prevent the apples from burning.

3. Let the applesauce cool. Then remove all the pieces of skin.

4. Gently chop to desired chunkiness.

5. Fill each piecrust with applesauce—1 heaping tablespoon per crust. Serve warm or cold.

*You may prefer to skip the pie crust and simply enjoy 3 to 4 heaping tablespoons of plain apple-sauce.

Creamy Pumpkin Pie

Serves 8

A citrusy crust made with gingersnaps and graham crackers perfectly complements the creamy, cinnamon-perfumed filling. This pie tastes great year-round, but it's an especially nice way to end a holiday meal. You can refrigerate leftovers (if there are any!).

CRUST

12 low-fat graham crackers, crushed

15 low-fat gingersnaps, crushed

2 tablespoons corn syrup

2 tablespoons orange juice

2 tablespoons diet margarine

FILLING

1 sixteen-ounce can pumpkin

3 egg whites

1 cup fat-free evaporated milk

¼ cup firmly packed brown sugar

¼ cup Splenda

1 teaspoon ground cinnamon

1 teaspoon ground ginger

¼ teaspoon ground nutmeg

¼ teaspoon ground cloves
½ teaspoon vanilla extract

TOPPING
8 tablespoons fat-free whipped topping

1. Preheat the oven to 350°.

2. Prepare the crust: In a medium bowl, combine all the crust ingredients and mix thoroughly. Press the mixture evenly into a deep 9-inch pie pan. Bake for 10 minutes. Remove to a rack to cool. Increase the oven heat to 450°.

3. Prepare the filling: In a large bowl, with the electric mixer set on medium speed, beat together all the filling ingredients for 2 minutes, or until smooth. Pour the filling into the prepared pie crust.

4. Bake the pie for 10 minutes on the center rack of the oven. Lower the oven temperature to 325° and bake for 50 to 55 minutes, until the center is fairly firm. Remove the pie to a rack to cool. Garnish each slice with 1 tablespoon fat-free whipped topping.

NUTRIENT ANALYSIS

◆ **1 SERVING = 1 SLICE (⅛ OF PIE)**

Calories: 191	Protein: 5.5 g	Carbohydrates: 36 g	Sugar: 16.8 g	Total fat: 3.7 g
Saturated fat: 1 g	Cholesterol: 1 mg	Sodium: 230 mg	Fiber: 2.3 g	Calcium: 144 mg
Potassium: 329 mg	Vitamin A (beta-carotene): 12,840 IU			

Ice Cream Berry Pie

Serves 8

This fun dessert for kids of all ages combines such favorites as ice cream, sandwich cookies, chocolate syrup, and fresh strawberries. Plan to make the pie at least 4 hours in advance so it has time to freeze.

4 cups low-fat vanilla ice cream or frozen yogurt (any brand fewer than 120 calories per ½ cup)
Oreo pie crust
2 cups sliced strawberries
¼ cup light chocolate Hershey's syrup

1. Let the ice cream thaw until it is soft and mushy. Spoon it into the Oreo piecrust and smooth the top. Cover with plastic pie top and tin foil and freeze for at least 4 hours.

2. Decorate the top with sliced strawberries. Drizzle chocolate syrup over the strawberries.

NUTRIENT ANALYSIS

♦ **1 SERVING = 1 SLICE (⅛ OF PIE)**

Calories: 233	Protein: 4 g	Carbohydrates: 38 g	Sugar: 29 g	Total fat: 7.4 g
Saturated fat: 2 g	Cholesterol: 5 mg	Sodium: 188 mg	Fiber: 2.7 g	Calcium: 115 mg

Oreo Vanilla Pudding Pie

Serves 6

A terrific three-ingredient dessert that takes minutes to assemble, this should chill for an hour before you slice it. You can substitute chocolate or even butterscotch pudding for the vanilla.

1 package Jell-O vanilla instant pudding mix*
Oreo piecrust
2 cups skim milk

*For fewer calories, use "fat-free, sugar-free" pudding mix.

1. Make the pudding according to package directions, using skim milk.

2. When the pudding thickens, pour it into the Oreo piecrust.

3. Refrigerate for at least 1 hour before serving.

◆ **1 SERVING= 1 SLICE (⅙ OF PIE)**

| Calories: 226 | Protein: 3.7 g | Carbohydrates: 36 g | Sugar: 24 g | Total fat: 7 g |

| Saturated fat: 1.5 g | Cholesterol: 1.5 g | Sodium: 447 mg | Fiber: 0.5 g | Calcium: 111 mg |

Peanut Butter Pie

Serves 8

If you're like millions of grown-ups and peanut butter is still one of your favorite foods, try this cool, creamy, and very easy pie. Be sure to use natural peanut butter, which is free of extra sugar and preservatives, and make the dessert in advance so it has time to chill in the fridge.

1 package "fat-free, sugar-free" instant vanilla pudding mix
1 cup skim milk, cold
¼ cup natural peanut butter (natural peanut butter separates; mix peanuts and oil before you measure)
1 cup Cool Whip Lite, frozen
1 graham cracker piecrust, or 8 small individual piecrusts (any brand 140 calories or fewer per serving)

1. In a mixing bowl, combine the pudding mix with cold skim milk. Whip until the pudding thickens.

2. Add the peanut butter and continue to whip until the peanut butter is thoroughly mixed through. Fold in Cool Whip. Mix.

3. Pour the mixture evenly into the graham cracker piecrust. Refrigerate at least 5 hours, until the pie is firm.

◆ **1 SERVING = 1 SLICE (⅛ OF PIE)**

Calories: 228	Protein: 4 g	Carbohydrates: 26 g	Sugar: 13 g	Total fat: 12 g
Saturated fat: 3.3 g	Cholesterol: 0 mg	Sodium: 235 mg	Fiber: 1 g	Calcium: 51 mg

Chocolate Chip Meringues

Serves 8 (6 meringues each)

Pure white puffs speckled with chocolate chips—these addictive little cookies are easy to make and impressive to look at. To get maximum volume from the egg whites, be sure both your bowl and beaters are completely clean before starting this recipe.

3 egg whites
Pinch of salt
½ teaspoon cream of tartar
½ teaspoon vanilla extract
½ cup sugar
¼ cup Splenda
½ cup mini–chocolate chips
Cooking spray

1. Preheat the oven to 300°.

2. In a large bowl, beat the egg whites, salt, cream of tartar, and vanilla extract on high speed. When soft peaks form, add ¼ cup sugar and beat again. When stiff peaks form, add the remaining sugar and Splenda and beat for several seconds.

3. Stir in the chocolate chips.

4. Spray two cookie sheets with cooking spray. Drop the meringues by the teaspoon onto the baking sheets about 1½ inches apart.

5. Bake for 20 minutes, rotating the baking pans twice. Turn off the oven and prop open the door a crack. Let the meringues dry in the oven for another ½ hour. Remove the meringues from the oven and place them on a rack to cool completely.

NUTRIENT ANALYSIS

♦ **1 SERVING = 6 MERINGUES**

Calories: 109	Protein: 1.8 g	Carbohydrates: 20 g	Sugar: 18 g	Total fat: 3.2 g
Saturated fat: 2 g	Cholesterol: 0 mg	Sodium: 168 mg	Fiber: 1 g	Calcium: 19 mg

Fudgy Brownie Squares

....

Serves 8 (2 brownies each)

Rich yet light, these brownies have the slightest hint of mocha. Be sure not to overbake them or they will be dry, and wait until they are completely cool before dusting with confectioner's sugar.

Vegetable oil spray
4 tablespoons butter
¼ cup semisweet chocolate chips
¼ cup coffee-flavored liqueur
1½ teaspoons vanilla extract
¼ teaspoon almond extract
¾ cup all-purpose flour
¾ teaspoon baking powder
¼ cup unsweetened cocoa
¼ teaspoon salt
¼ cup plus 2 tablespoons dark brown sugar
¼ cup Splenda
1 egg
1 tablespoon confectioner's sugar

1. Preheat the oven to 350°. Spray an 8-inch-square baking pan with vegetable oil spray.

2. In small glass bowl, combine the butter and chocolate chips. Heat in the microwave for 2 minutes, or until melted. Stir and set aside to cool. When cool, stir in the coffee-flavored liqueur, vanilla extract, and almond extract.

3. Sift together the flour, baking powder, cocoa, and salt.

4. In mixing bowl, beat together the brown sugar, Splenda, and egg for 1 minute. Add the chocolate mixture and beat well. Add the flour mixture and beat until smooth.

5. Spoon and scrape the batter into the prepared pan. Bake for 20 minutes or until a toothpick inserted into the center comes out clean.

6. Let cool for 15 minutes. Sift the confectioner's sugar over the top. When completely cool, cut into 16 small brownies.

NUTRIENT ANALYSIS

◆ **1 SERVING = 2 BROWNIES**

Calories: 198	Protein: 3 g	Carbohydrates: 24 g	Sugar: 12 g	Total fat: 8 g
Saturated fat: 4.5 g	Cholesterol: 42 mg	Sodium: 180 mg	Fiber: 2 g	Calcium: 40 mg

Ice Cream Cookie Sandwiches

Serves 6

The classic ice cream sandwich gets a remake in this luscious dessert. Chocolate chip cookies hold the filling, and rainbow sprinkles lend a festive touch. Make them a few hours in advance so they have time to harden. Then wrap the sandwiches individually and store in the freezer for when you have an insatiable craving for something cold, creamy, and crunchy.

1 pint low-fat ice cream or frozen yogurt (flavor of your choice)
12 reduced-fat Chips Ahoy cookies
1 cup chocolate or rainbow sprinkles

1. Let the ice cream get soft enough to scoop easily.

2. Lay out 6 cookies bottom up. Top each with 1 large scoop of low-fat ice cream or frozen yogurt.

3. Top each cookie with another cookie and press down gently.

4. Place the sprinkles in a shallow bowl. Roll the sides of each ice cream cookie sandwich in the sprinkles.

6. Wrap in plastic wrap and freeze until ready to serve.

NUTRIENT ANALYSIS				
◆ 1 SERVING = 1 SANDWICH				
Calories: 166	Protein: 3 g	Carbohydrates: 27 g	Sugar: 17.9 g	Total fat: 5 g
Saturated fat: 1.6 g	Cholesterol: 3 mg	Sodium: 133 mg	Fiber: 1.3 g	Calcium: 73 mg

Rebecca's Oatmeal Chip Cookies

Makes 16 cookies

An old-fashioned cookie jar treat bursting with chocolate chips, these addictive cookies will be a favorite with your kids, too. Use the quick-cooking oatmeal, not the instant, sweetened variety.

1/3 cup unsweetened applesauce
1/2 cup + 2 tablespoons Splenda
1 tablespoon canola oil
2 egg whites
1 teaspoon vanilla extract
1/2 teaspoon ground allspice
1/4 teaspoon salt
1/2 teaspoon baking soda
1 tablespoon cinnamon

1½ cups quick-cooking oatmeal, dry
½ cup semisweet chocolate chips
Cooking spray

1. Preheat the oven to 375°.

2. In a large mixing bowl, combine the applesauce, Splenda, and canola oil. Mix in the egg whites and vanilla extract.

3. In a separate bowl, mix together the allspice, salt, baking soda, and cinnamon. Add to the applesauce mixture.

4. Gradually add the oatmeal and chocolate chips and mix thoroughly.

5. Spray a cookie sheet with cooking spray. Use a tablespoon to create 16 round cookies. Flatten them slightly with spoon. Bake for 10 to 12 minutes.

NUTRIENT ANALYSIS

◆ **1 SERVING = 2 COOKIES**

Calories: 140	Protein: 3.4 g	Carbohydrates: 20 g	Sugar: 7 g	Total fat: 6 g
Saturated fat: 2 g	Cholesterol: 0 mg	Sodium: 168 mg	Fiber: 2.4 g	Calcium: 52 mg

Stovetop S'mores

Serves 1

You don't need to be a Girl Scout and you don't need a campfire to make my version of the classic kids' dessert. Enjoy them with your children on a snowy winter night, or go ahead and indulge with a group of adults! Just make sure you don't eat the leftover chocolate squares.

1 graham cracker broken into 4 small strips
2 marshmallows
1 Hershey's milk chocolate bar (1.55 ounces) broken into 12 small rectangles

1. Roast the marshmallows over an open flame on the stove.

2. Place the marshmallows on 1 piece of graham cracker.

3. Place 2 small pieces of chocolate on top of the marshmallow.

4. Cover with 1 more piece of graham cracker to form a sandwich.

NUTRIENT ANALYSIS

♦ **1 SERVING = 1 S'MORE SANDWICH**

Calories: 202	Protein: 2.7 g	Carbohydrates: 37 g	Sugar: 16 g	Total fat: 5 g
Saturated fat: 1.8 g	Cholesterol: 0 mg	Sodium: 182 mg	Fiber: 1 g	Calcium: 19 mg

Chocolate Mousse

Serves 4

My version of the classic French dessert, this chocolate lover's dream is extra creamy and smooth. For easier mixing, thaw the Cool Whip before adding it to the recipe. And be sure to save ½ cup so you can use it to garnish each serving. This tastes great frozen too!

1½ cups skim milk, cold
1 package Jell-O "sugar-free, fat-free" chocolate pudding mix
1½ cups Cool Whip Lite

1. In a mixing bowl, first pour in the cold skim milk and then add the chocolate pudding mix. Whip with a wire whisk or electric mixer for 5 minutes until the pudding thickens.

2. Add 1 cup Cool Whip to the pudding mixture and gently whip.

3. Divide the mousse into four serving dishes. Chill in the refrigerator for 30 minutes or more. Top each with a dollop of Cool Whip.

Microwave Chocolate Pudding

Serves 6

This super easy, superfast dessert is meant for diehard chocoholics in need of a quick fix. It's smooth and rich—a perfect snack for when you want to unwind in front of the television at night. As an added benefit, this pudding is a good source of calcium and vitamin D.

12 tablespoons sugar
½ cup unsweetened cocoa
4 tablespoons cornstarch
3 cups 1% low-fat milk
1½ teaspoons vanilla extract
Reduced-fat whipped cream or topping (such as Cool Whip Lite)

1. In large mixing bowl, stir together the sugar, cocoa, and cornstarch. Gradually add the milk and stir with a whisk to blend. Microwave on high for 6 minutes, stirring every 2 minutes. Microwave on medium for 3 minutes, stirring every minute, or until thick. Remove and add the vanilla. Stir.

2. Cover and chill for 30 minutes or more. Serve each portion with 2 tablespoons of reduced-fat whipped cream.

BlueEarth's Pineapple Lemongrass Skewers

Serves 4

This exotic, cooling dessert with flavors reminiscent of Thai cuisine is garnished with sorbet or frozen yogurt and plenty of chopped fresh mint. To ensure that the skewers don't darken or burn during the grilling process, be sure to soak them in water for about 30 minutes before starting this recipe.

2 cups fresh pineapple cut into 1-inch cubes (or canned pineapple in extra-light syrup, rinsed and drained)
4 six-inch stalks lemongrass
1 tablespoon vanilla extract
1 teaspoon spiced rum
1 tablespoon thinly sliced mint, for garnish

1. Skewer and marinate the pineapple in 4 equal servings with all the ingredients except the mint for 30 minutes.

2. Heat a grill or grill pan to high. Grill the skewers on all sides until lightly browned, approximately 3 minutes total.

3. Serve warm with 1 small scoop (½ cup) sorbet or low-fat yogurt. Garnish with fresh mint.

◆ **1 SERVING = 1 SKEWER WITH ½ CUP SORBET**

Calories: 178	Protein: 0.5 g	Carbohydrates: 42 g	Sugar: 35 g	Total fat: 0 g
Saturated fat: 0 g	Cholesterol: 0 mg	Sodium: 1.6 mg	Fiber: 3 g	Calcium: 52 mg

Frosty Apple Smoothie

Serves 6

This tastes like a gently spiced cider milkshake, and it's pretty to look at, too, when sprinkled with fresh nutmeg. For best results, use a blender to whip up all the ingredients. This smoothie is best when made just before serving.

1 pint low-fat vanilla ice cream (any brand 120 or fewer calories per ½-cup serving)
24 ounces apple cider
1 cup ice cubes or crushed ice
Nutmeg (optional)
Cinnamon (optional)

Combine the ice cream, apple cider, and ice in a blender. Mix until smooth. Pour into glasses and sprinkle with either nutmeg or cinnamon.

NUTRIENT ANALYSIS

◆ **1 SERVING = 1 CUP**

Calories: 116	Protein: 2 g	Carbohydrates: 13.5 g	Sugar: 11 g	Total fat: 1.4 g
Saturated fat: 0.7 g	Cholesterol: 3 mg	Sodium: 33 mg	Fiber: 1 g	Calcium: 80 mg

Cranberry Couscous

Serves 3

When you want a warm, filling snack, or a side starch to a low-calorie dinner, this is the perfect recipe. It couldn't be easier, since couscous is ready in just 5 minutes, and the tangy flavor and pretty color of the dried cranberries add interest. Be sure to use plain couscous, not one that's flavored with herbs or garlic.

2 cups fat-free chicken broth
1 tablespoon reduced-fat, soft tub margarine
1 cup dry, plain quick-cooking couscous
3 tablespoons dried cranberries

1. In a saucepan, bring the chicken broth and margarine to a boil.

2. Add the couscous, cover, and remove from heat. Wait 5 minutes and then fluff with a spoon.

3. Add the cranberries and mix thoroughly.

NUTRIENT ANALYSIS

♦ **1 SERVING = ¾ CUP**

| Calories: 213 | Protein: 7.5 g | Carbohydrates: 41 g | Sugar: 4 g | Total fat: 1.7 g |
| Saturated fat: 0 g | Cholesterol: 0 mg | Sodium: 300 mg | Fiber: 2.6 g | Calcium: 21 mg |

Oven-Baked French Fries

Serves 2

There's no need to visit a fast-food drive-through when the urge for crisp, golden brown french fries strikes. You'll never miss the fat in my irresistible version—and they're clearly much better for your heart, too!

2 medium potatoes, approximately 7 ounces each
Cooking spray
½ teaspoon salt
*Optional spices

1. Preheat the oven to 375°.

2. Slice the potatoes into thin strips, then cut those strips in half. Aim for fries to be approximately ¼ inch thick.

3. Coat a baking sheet with cooking spray and lay out the potato strips. Spray the potato strips with cooking spray and sprinkle with salt. *You may also add optional spices.

4. Bake for 20 minutes. Then set the oven to broil and cook for an additional 5 to 10 minutes (depending on how browned and crunchy you prefer your fries).

NUTRIENT ANALYSIS

♦ **1 SERVING = ABOUT 15 FRIES**

Calories: 220	Protein: 4.6 g	Carbohydrates: 50 g	Sugar: 3 g	Total fat: 0 g
Saturated fat: 0 g	Cholesterol: 0 mg	Sodium: 597 mg	Fiber: 5 g	Calcium: 20 mg
Potassium: 844 mg	Vitamin C: 20 mg			

Garlic Smashed Potatoes

Serves 6

This is the way that spuds were meant to be eaten: creamy, fluffy, and lightly flavored with garlic. You won't miss the butter in this homey dish, but you will taste the tangy buttermilk. Besides stirring roasted, pureed garlic into the cooked potatoes, you boil the potatoes with garlic, too.

1 whole head garlic plus 3 cloves
2 pounds (about 6) large red potatoes
7 tablespoons buttermilk
2 tablespoons reduced-fat, soft tub margarine
Salt and freshly ground black pepper

1. Preheat the oven to 325°.

2. Cut the top third off the head of garlic and discard. Place trimmed garlic in a small baking dish and add water to partially cover. Cover with foil and bake for 45 to 55 minutes, until the garlic is very soft.

3. Peel the 3 cloves of garlic. Peel the potatoes and cut them into large chunks. In a large pot of boiling, lightly salted water, cook the potatoes with the garlic over medium heat for 10 minutes, or until soft.

4. Drain off the water, then shake the pan over low heat until the potatoes look dry. With a potato masher, mash the hot potatoes, trying to smooth out all the lumps.

5. In a small saucepan, heat the buttermilk until very hot. Stir in the margarine. Add the hot buttermilk mixture to the potatoes and whip the potatoes with a fork. Stir in salt and pepper to taste.

6. Squeeze the pulp out of the roasted garlic and add it to the mashed potatoes. Mix well.

Guacamole

Serves 5

For the best flavor, choose black, pebbly-textured Hass avocados for this authentic south-of-the-border dip. Be sure to chop the onion and garlic very finely, and make this just a couple of hours before you plan to serve it. Great for a party or special dinner.

4 medium ripe avocados
½ cup chopped onion
½ cup chopped tomato
2 cloves garlic, finely chopped
Juice of 1 fresh lime
Salt and freshly ground black pepper

1. Scoop out the insides of the avocados into a bowl. Mash with a fork until smooth.

2. Add the onion, tomato, garlic, and lime juice. Mix. Add salt and pepper to taste.

Hot Artichoke Dip

Serves 4

A wonderfully festive dip for a party, this tastes best piping hot. If you're planning to put it out for guests at a buffet, spoon into a fondue dish and place it over a flame. Be sure to serve with lots of fresh, colorful cut-up veggies.

2 pitas, cut into 8 wedges each
Cooking spray
1 teaspoon sea salt
¾ cup low-fat mayonnaise (any brand with 25 calories or fewer per tablespoon)
½ cup freshly grated Parmesan cheese
1 fourteen-ounce can artichoke hearts, drained and chopped
2 scallions, finely chopped
Carrots, red pepper strips, cucumbers, raw mushrooms, broccoli florets

1. Preheat the oven to 375°. Spray the pita wedges with cooking oil and dust them with salt. Toast in the oven for 5 minutes, or until golden. Reduce the oven temperature to 350°.

2. In a small bowl, stir together the mayonnaise and Parmesan. Stir in the artichoke hearts and scallions. Mix well.

3. Spoon the mixture into a small casserole dish and bake for 25 minutes, or until hot. Serve with the toasted pita wedges and the raw vegetables.

NUTRIENT ANALYSIS

♦ **1 SERVING= ¼ CUP DIP, 4 PITA WEDGES, AND VEGGIES**

Calories: 228	Protein: 11 g	Carbohydrates: 34 g	Sugar: 7.6 g	Total fat: 4.4 g
Saturated fat: 2.5 g	Cholesterol: 9.8 mg	Sodium: 1592 mg	Fiber: 2 g	Calcium: 215 mg

My Fun Foods chapter ends these recipes on a sweet (and salty) note. But your commitment to a new, healthier way of eating doesn't stop here. I'm confident that, armed with the tools you've gained by reading these pages, you'll make a decision to follow a healthier lifestyle that involves maintaining your goal weight while eating well.

You're now skilled in deciphering a nutrition label and eyeballing the correct portion size. And you know where to shop in the supermarket for the best buys, and how to prepare meat, poultry, fish, and produce for maximum flavor and minimal calories. The final chapter offers valuable assistance for when you plan meals and special menus. In fact, you'll find two complete weeks' worth of menus that you can either follow to the letter, or mix and match according to your likes and dislikes. It may help eliminate anxiety about what foods go best with each other, give you ideas for what to serve your family for a special occasion, and, most of all, keep you motivated with a collection of interesting and varied menus.

I know that you will find continued success not just in keeping off the weight, but in feeling good about yourself and satisfied with the meals you eat. Above all, I wish you a positive relationship with food and a lifetime of good health.

Ten

Mixing It Up:
The Fourteen-Day Menu Plan
(plus The Vegetarian Diet Plan)

The Fourteen Day-Menu Plan

If you like things precisely laid out, this two-week plan is for you. I provide breakfasts, lunches, dinners, and snacks, all carefully calculated to give you maximum taste, variety, and satisfaction while helping you to painlessly meet your weight-loss goals. Each recipe contains the perfect balance of nutrients so that you'll feel energetic throughout the day and not feel hungry between meals/snacks. You may want to follow this diet 100 percent, or you may decide to use just part of the plan and to mix it up with another calorie-controlled weight-loss plan—your own, my original *90/10 Weight-Loss Plan*, or another one you're following. Either way, you'll be pleased with the results, as this is a way of eating that will soon have you looking and feeling better.

You may repeat this diet plan for as long as you like. And because all recipes in a category are calorically equivalent, you may mix and match breakfasts with breakfasts, lunches with lunches, snacks with snacks, dinners with dinners, and fun foods with fun foods. Also, when you prepare a recipe, be sure to stick with the portion size listed underneath your personal calorie level—and enjoy all of the accompaniments that come with it. If you decide to skip the fun food/dessert on any given day, you're entitled to add back 250 calories' worth of healthier alternatives into your daily plan (extra fruit, nuts, lean protein, or perhaps a bigger portion of your fish with dinner).

On the plan, as with all weight-loss plans, it's a good idea to drink plenty of water. Feel free to drink other noncaloric beverages during the day if you like them. You may have diet beverages and unsweetened iced tea, and you may sweeten both tea and coffee with artificial sweeteners in moderation.

I also recommend that both men and women take a regular one-a-day multivitamin/mineral that supplies 100 percent of the recommended dietary allowances. Try to take the supplement with food and at the same time each day, so that it becomes a habit. Keep in mind that most women should also be taking separate calcium supplements in the form of calcium carbonate or calcium citrate (with added vitamin D and magnesium). Your body can't use more than 600 milligrams of calcium at a time, so if you are taking more, take one pill in the morning and one in the evening. And be sure you don't overdo vitamin D, as it can become toxic when taken in large amounts. Do not exceed a total of 1,000 IU from both your multivitamin/mineral and calcium supplements.

YOUR CALORIE BREAKDOWNS AT A GLANCE

Meal	1,200 Plan	1,400 Plan	1,600 Plan	1,800 Plan	2,000 Plan
Breakfast	200	250	250	300	350
Lunch	300	350	400	500	500
Snack	100	100	150	200	250
Dinner	350	450	550	550	650
Fun Food	250	250	250	250	250

Day 1

BREAKFAST
Cheddar Mushroom Omelet (page 79)

LUNCH
Cape Cod Tuna Salad (page 119)

SNACK
1,200-calorie plan: 10 whole cashews or 14 almonds
1,400-calorie plan: 10 whole cashews or 14 almonds

1,600-calorie plan: 15 whole cashews or 20 almonds
1,800-calorie plan: 20 whole cashews or 28 almonds
2,000-calorie plan: 25 whole cashews or 35 almonds

DINNER
Tex-Mex Turkey Burger (page 149)

FUN FOOD
Oven-Baked French Fries *with dinner* (page 287)
Or
BlueEarth's Pineapple Lemongrass Skewers with sorbet (page 284)

Day 2

BREAKFAST
Low-Fat Granola (page 93)

LUNCH
Boston Crab Salad Triangles (page 117)

SNACK
1,200-calorie plan: Apple
1,400-calorie plan: Apple
1,600-calorie plan: Apple + 2 level teaspoons peanut butter (or 1 slice fat-free cheese)
1,800-calorie plan: Apple + 1 level tablespoon peanut butter (or 2 slices fat-free cheese)
2,000-calorie plan: Apple + 1 level tablespoon peanut butter (or 2 slices fat-free cheese) + peach,
    plum, or orange

DINNER
Chicken Piccata (page 202)

FUN FOOD
Angel Food Cake with Fresh Berries (page 267)

Day 3

BREAKFAST
Strawberry Yogurt Parfait (page 97)

LUNCH
Black Bean and Spinach Burrito (page 111)

SNACK
1,200-calorie plan: Turkey roll-ups: 2 ounces sliced turkey breast with mustard + cucumber slices

1,400-calorie plan: Turkey roll-ups: 2 ounces sliced turkey breast with mustard + cucumber slices

1,600-calorie plan: Turkey roll-ups: 3 ounces sliced turkey breast with mustard + cucumber slices

1,800-calorie plan: Turkey roll-ups: 4 ounces (¼ pound) sliced turkey breast with mustard + cucumber slices

2,000-calorie plan: Turkey roll-ups: 4 ounces (¼ pound) sliced turkey breast with mustard + cucumber slices and 15 cherry tomatoes

DINNER
Zuppa di Pesce (page 225)

FUN FOOD
Chocolate Chip Meringues (page 277)

Day 4

BREAKFAST
Vegetable Frittata (page 81)

LUNCH
Red Lentil and Bulgar Pilaf (page 123)

SNACK
1,200-calorie plan: 1 rice cake topped with 1 slice low-fat or fat-free cheese and tomato

1,400-calorie plan: 1 rice cake topped with 1 slice low-fat or fat-free cheese and tomato

1,600-calorie plan: 1 rice cake topped with 1 slice low-fat or fat-free cheese and tomato; ½ grapefruit, 1 orange, 1 peach, or ¼ cantaloupe

1,800-calorie plan: 2 rice cakes topped with 2 slices low-fat or fat-free cheese and tomato + 8 baby carrots

2,000-calorie plan: 3 rice cakes topped with 3 slices low-fat cheese or fat-free cheese and tomato

DINNER
Shrimp Creole (page 230)

FUN FOOD
Chocolate Mousse (page 282)

Day 5

BREAKFAST
Grandma's Cheese Pancakes (page 71)

LUNCH
Egg White Vegetable Dijonnaise (page 113)

SNACK
1,200-calorie plan: Skim café latte (optional, 1 packet Splenda or Equal)

1,400-calorie plan: Skim café latte (optional, 1 packet Splenda or Equal)

1,600-calorie plan: Skim café latte (optional, 1 packet Splenda or Equal) + 1 peach, plum, orange, small apple, or 1 cup whole strawberries

1,800-calorie plan: Skim café latte (optional, 1 packet Splenda or Equal) + ½ cantaloupe or 1 cup fresh fruit salad

2,000-calorie plan: Skim café latte (optional, 1 packet Splenda or Equal) + ½ cantaloupe or 1 cup fresh fruit salad + 7 almonds

DINNER
Herb-Marinated Flank Steak (page 153)

Garlic Smashed Potatoes *with dinner* (page 288)

Day 6

BREAKFAST
Blueberry Yogurt Pancakes (page 69)

LUNCH
Baba Ghanouj (page 103)

SNACK
1,200-calorie plan: ½ cup 1 percent low-fat cottage cheese (optional, cinnamon) + celery sticks
1,400-calorie plan: ½ cup 1 percent low-fat cottage cheese (optional, cinnamon) + celery sticks
1,600-calorie plan: ¾ cup low-fat cottage cheese (optional, cinnamon) + celery sticks
1,800-calorie plan: 1 cup low-fat cottage cheese + ½ cup fresh pineapple or blueberries
2,000-calorie plan: 1 cup 1 percent low-fat cottage cheese + 1 cup fresh pineapple or blueberries

DINNER
Spicy Jambalaya (page 169)

FUN FOOD
Fudgy Brownie Squares (page 278)

Day 7

BREAKFAST
Apple Cinnamon Crepes (page 67)

LUNCH
Southwestern Chicken Soup (page 101)

SNACK

1,200-calorie plan: 1 level tablespoon peanut butter (or 2 tablespoons low-fat cream cheese) spread over 1 stalk celery

1,400-calorie plan: 1 level tablespoon peanut butter (or 2 tablespoons low-fat cream cheese) spread over 1 stalk celery

1,600-calorie plan: 1½ level tablespoons peanut butter (or 3 tablespoons low-fat cream cheese) spread over 1 stalk celery

1,800-calorie plan: 2 level tablespoons peanut butter (or 4 tablespoons low-fat cream cheese) spread over 2 stalks celery

2,000-calorie plan: 2 level tablespoons peanut butter (or 4 tablespoons low-fat cream cheese) spread over 2 stalks celery + 1 peach, plum, or orange

DINNER

Extra-Lean Turkey Chili (page 139)

FUN FOOD

Ice Cream Cookie Sandwich (page 279)

Day 8

BREAKFAST

Scrambled Egg Whites, Lox, and Tomato (page 83)

LUNCH

Hummus (page 105)

SNACK

1,200-calorie plan: Turkey roll-ups: 2 ounces sliced turkey breast with mustard + cucumber slices

1,400-calorie plan: Turkey roll-ups: 2 ounces sliced turkey breast with mustard + cucumber slices

1,600-calorie plan: Turkey roll-ups: 3 ounces sliced turkey breast with mustard + cucumber slices

1,800-calorie plan: Turkey roll-ups: 4 ounces (¼ pound) sliced turkey breast with mustard + cucumber slices

2,000-calorie plan: Turkey roll-ups: 4 ounces (¼ pound) sliced turkey breast with mustard + cucumber slices and 15 cherry tomatoes

DINNER
Apple Dijon–Encrusted Loin of Pork (page 211)

FUN FOOD
Strawberry-Topped Cheesecake (page 269)

Day 9

BREAKFAST
Applesauce Muffins (page 85)
Or
Pumpkin Muffins (page 89)
Or
Oatmeal Berry Muffins (page 87)

LUNCH
Cape Cod Tuna Salad (page 119)
Or
Boston Crab Salad Triangles (page 117)
Or
Egg White Vegetable Dijonnaise (page 113)

SNACK
1,200-calorie plan: 2 level tablespoons Hummus (page 105) + 8 baby carrots
1,400-calorie plan: 2 level tablespoons Hummus (page 105) + 8 baby carrots
1,600-calorie plan: 3 level tablespoons Hummus (page 105) + 16 baby carrots
1,800-calorie plan: 4 level tablespoons Hummus (page 105) + 16 baby carrots
2,000-calorie plan: 6 level tablespoons Hummus (page 105) + 16 baby carrots

DINNER
Veal Marsala with Spaghetti Squash (page 194)

FUN FOOD
Microwave Chocolate Pudding (page 283)

Day 10

BREAKFAST
Cottage Cheese Rice Bowl (page 77)

LUNCH
Grilled Vegetable Sandwich (page 115)

SNACK
1,200-calorie plan: 6 ounces nonfat flavored yogurt (any brand 100 calories or fewer)
1,400-calorie plan: 6 ounces nonfat flavored yogurt (any brand 100 calories or fewer)
1,600-calorie plan: 6 ounces nonfat flavored yogurt (any brand 100 calories or fewer) + 2 tablespoons low-fat granola or wheat germ
1,800-calorie plan: 8 ounces nonfat flavored yogurt (any brand 150 calories or fewer) + 2 tablespoons low-fat granola or wheat germ
2,000-calorie plan: 8 ounces nonfat flavored yogurt (any brand 150 calories or fewer) + 2 tablespoons low-fat granola or wheat germ + 16 baby carrots

DINNER
Southwestern Turkey Meat Loaf (page 147)

FUN FOOD
Stovetop S'more (page 281)

Day 11

BREAKFAST
Pineapple Cheese Pancakes (page 73)

LUNCH
Cool Tabbouleh with Mint (page 121)

1,200-calorie plan: 2 slices 40-calorie whole wheat bread, toasted (or 70-calorie whole wheat pita) + 1 level teaspoon peanut butter (or 2 teaspoons low-fat cream cheese) and 1 teaspoon sugar-free jam

1,400-calorie plan: 2 slices 40-calorie whole wheat bread, toasted (or 70-calorie whole wheat pita) + 1 level teaspoon peanut butter (or 2 teaspoons low-fat cream cheese) and 1 teaspoon sugar-free jam

1,600-calorie plan: 2 slices 40-calorie whole wheat bread, toasted (or 70-calorie whole wheat pita) + 2 level teaspoons peanut butter (or 4 teaspoons low-fat cream cheese) and 1–2 teaspoons sugar-free jam

1,800-calorie plan: 2 slices 40-calorie whole wheat bread, toasted (or 70-calorie whole wheat pita) + 2 level teaspoons peanut butter (or 4 teaspoons low-fat cream cheese) and 1–2 teaspoons sugar-free jam + 1 orange or ½ grapefruit

2,000-calorie plan: 2 slices 40-calorie whole wheat bread, toasted (or 70-calorie whole wheat pita) + 2 level teaspoons peanut butter (or 4 teaspoons low-fat cream cheese) and 1–2 teaspoons sugar-free jam + apple, pear, or banana

DINNER
Microwave Stuffed Peppers (page 141)

FUN FOOD
Chunky Applesauce Pie (page 272)

Day 12

BREAKFAST
Fruity Tofu Yogurt Shake (page 95)

LUNCH
Red Lentil Dip with Crudités and Pita Wedges (page 107)

SNACK
1,200-calorie plan: 10 whole cashews or 14 almonds
1,400-calorie plan: 10 whole cashews or 14 almonds
1,600-calorie plan: 15 whole cashews or 20 almonds

1,800-calorie plan: 20 whole cashews or 28 almonds

2,000-calorie plan: 25 whole cashews or 35 almonds

DINNER
Chicken Florentine (page 200)

FUN FOOD
Lemon Ginger Pudding Cake (page 268)

Day 13

BREAKFAST
Strawberry Oat Pancakes (page 75)

LUNCH
Three-Cheese Quesadilla (page 109)

SNACK

1,200-calorie plan: Smoothie: ¾ cup skim milk blended with ½–1 cup frozen whole strawberries (optional, ¼ cup crushed ice and 1 packet Splenda or Equal)

1,400-calorie plan: Smoothie: ¾ cup skim milk blended with ½–1 cup frozen whole strawberries (optional, ¼ cup crushed ice and 1 packet Splenda or Equal)

1,600-calorie plan: Smoothie: 1 cup skim milk blended with 1 cup frozen whole strawberries (optional, ¼ cup crushed ice and 1 packet Splenda or Equal)

1,800-calorie plan: Smoothie: 1 cup skim milk blended with 1 cup frozen whole strawberries and ½ cup fresh blueberries or ½ banana (optional, ¼ cup crushed ice and 1 packet Splenda or Equal)

2,000-calorie plan: Smoothie: 1 cup skim milk blended with 1 cup frozen whole strawberries and ½ cup fresh blueberries or ½ banana (optional, ¼ cup crushed ice and 1 packet Splenda or Equal) + 16 baby carrots

DINNER
Asian Citrus Salmon Steak (page 159)

Cranberry Couscous *with dinner* (page 286)

Or

Chocolate Mousse (page 282)

Day 14

BREAKFAST
Cranberry Pecan Scones (page 91)

LUNCH
Boston Crab Salad Triangles (page 117)

SNACK
1,200-calorie plan: 1 banana (frozen or room temperature)
1,400-calorie plan: 1 banana (frozen or room temperature)
1,600-calorie plan: 1 banana (frozen or room temperature) + 7 whole almonds
1,800-calorie plan: 1 banana (frozen or room temperature) + 14 whole almonds
2,000-calorie plan: 1 banana (frozen or room temperature) + 20 whole almonds

DINNER
Slow-Cooker Beef Stroganoff (page 155)

FUN FOOD
Ice Cream Berry Pie (page 274)

The Vegetarian Diet Plan

If you're a vegan (a strict vegetarian who doesn't eat *anything* from an animal, including cow's milk, yogurt, or eggs), a less radical vegetarian who simply avoids meat, fish, and poultry, or just someone who wants to try something new, here's a seven-day diet that will enable you to lose weight, feel great, and still avoid all animal products. If you're feeling really motivated, you can dive right in and give this plan 100 percent of your effort. However, preparing the recipes can certainly take up considerable time and energy. Instead, you may decide to use just part of this plan and mix it up with another calorie-controlled weight-loss regimen—my original *90/10 Weight-Loss Plan*, your own creation, or another program you're following. However you decide to tailor it, if you follow the plan, you'll be thrilled with the results.

I've manipulated the recipe combinations to provide you with adequate nutrition and protein so you always feel satisfied, never deprived. Before you get started, here are a few important cooking tips specifically for vegetarians.

- In all recipes, substitute an equal amount of low-fat soy milk or rice milk for cow's milk.
- Substitute the same amount of low-fat soy yogurt for regular yogurt.
- Substitute the same amount of soy cheese for regular low-fat cheese.
- Substitute the same amount of soy sour cream for regular low-fat sour cream.
- When subbing tofu for meat, chicken, or fish, use *twice as much* tofu (when comparing in ounces).

Substitutions for eggs are tricky because there is no substitute I feel is appropriate in many of the breakfast recipes. For vegans, I've placed an asterisk next to all egg-containing recipes. Instead of making a dish with eggs to start off your morning, you may want to consider these simple breakfast ideas instead:

- High-fiber cereal with low-fat soy milk and fruit
- Soy yogurt with slivered almonds and fresh fruit
- Whole-grain toast topped with peanut or soy nut butter and fresh fruit

Of course, you still have to calculate the right amount of calories for your personal breakfast—all of that how-to information is in Chapter 1 and in the box below. Read the labels on packages and containers to make sure you're placing the right amount of food in your bowl or on your plate.

You may repeat this seven-day rotation diet plan for as many weeks as you like. And because all recipes in a category are calorically equivalent, you may mix and match breakfasts with breakfasts, lunches with lunches, snacks with snacks, dinners with dinners, and fun foods with fun foods. If you decide to skip the fun food/dessert on any given day, that's fine. You're entitled to add 250 calories' worth of healthier alternatives back into your daily plan (extra fruit, a soy protein shake, nuts, a protein bar). Also, when you prepare a recipe, be sure to stick with the portion size listed underneath your personal calorie level—and enjoy all of the accompaniments that come with it.

As for what to drink, my first choice is water, but feel free to drink other noncaloric beverages during the day. You may have diet beverages and unsweetened iced tea, and you may sweeten both tea and coffee with artificial sweeteners in moderation.

I also recommend that both men and women take a regular one-a-day multivitamin/mineral that supplies 100 percent of the recommended dietary allowances. Try to take the supplement with food and at the same time each day, so that it becomes a habit. Keep in mind that most women should also be taking separate calcium supplements in the form of calcium carbonate or calcium citrate (with added vitamin D and magnesium). Your body can't use more than 600 milligrams of calcium at a time, so if you are taking more, take one pill in the morning and one in the evening. And be sure you don't overdo vitamin D, as it can become toxic when taken in large amounts. Do not exceed a total of 1,000 IU from both your multivitamin/mineral and calcium supplements.

YOUR CALORIE BREAKDOWNS AT A GLANCE

Meal	1,200 Plan	1,400 Plan	1,600 Plan	1,800 Plan	2,000 Plan
Breakfast	200	250	250	300	350
Lunch	300	350	400	500	500
Snack	100	100	150	200	250
Dinner	350	450	550	550	650
Fun Food	250	250	250	250	250

Day 1

BREAKFAST
*Applesauce Muffins (page 85)

LUNCH
Red Lentil and Bulgar Pilaf (page 123)

SNACK
1,200-calorie plan: 10 whole cashews or 14 almonds
1,400-calorie plan: 10 whole cashews or 14 almonds
1,600-calorie plan: 15 whole cashews or 20 almonds
1,800-calorie plan: 20 whole cashews or 28 almonds
2,000-calorie plan: 25 whole cashews or 35 almonds

DINNER
Vegetarian Lentil Chili (page 232)

FUN FOOD
*Angel Food Cake with Fresh Berries (page 267)

Day 2

BREAKFAST
Fruity Tofu Yogurt Shake (page 95)

LUNCH
Black Bean and Spinach Burrito (page 111)

SNACK
1,200-calorie plan: 2 level tablespoons Hummus (page 105) + 8 baby carrots
1,400-calorie plan: 2 level tablespoons Hummus (page 105) + 8 baby carrots
1,600-calorie plan: 3 level tablespoons Hummus (page 105) + 16 baby carrots
1,800-calorie plan: 4 level tablespoons Hummus (page 105) + 16 baby carrots
2,000-calorie plan: 6 level tablespoons Hummus (page 105) + 16 baby carrots

DINNER
Cold Sesame Noodles (page 173)

FUN FOOD
BlueEarth's Pineapple Lemongrass Skewers, with sorbet (page 284)

Day 3

BREAKFAST
Low-Fat Granola (page 93)

LUNCH
Baba Ghanouj (page 103)

SNACK
1,200-calorie plan: 1 level tablespoon peanut butter (or soy nut butter) spread over 1 stalk celery
1,400-calorie plan: 1 level tablespoon peanut butter (or soy nut butter) spread over 1 stalk celery
1,600-calorie plan: 1½ level tablespoons peanut butter (or soy nut butter) spread over 1 stalk celery
1,800-calorie plan: 2 level tablespoons peanut butter (or soy nut butter) spread over 1–2 stalks celery
2,000-calorie plan: 2 level tablespoons peanut butter (or soy nut butter) spread over 1–2 stalk celery + 1 peach, plum, or orange.

DINNER
Honey Ginger Stir-Fry (substitute tofu for chicken) (page 135)

FUN FOOD
*Lemon Ginger Pudding Cake (page 268)

Day 4

BREAKFAST
*Blueberry Yogurt Pancakes (page 69)

LUNCH
Hummus (page 105)

SNACK

1,200-calorie plan: 1 banana (frozen or at room temperature)

1,400-calorie plan: 1 banana (frozen or at room temperature)

1,600-calorie plan: 1 banana (frozen or at room temperature) + 7 whole almonds

1,800-calorie plan: 1 banana (frozen or at room temperature) + 14 whole almonds

2,000-calorie plan: 1 banana (frozen or at room temperature) + 20 whole almonds

DINNER

Black Bean Soup with Sherry and Garlic (page 181)

FUN FOOD

Frosty Apple Smoothie (substitute vanilla Tofutti for ice cream) (page 285)

Day 5

BREAKFAST

*Cranberry Pecan Scones (page 91)

LUNCH

Cool Tabbouleh with Mint (page 121)

SNACK

1,200-calorie plan: 1 cup boiled edamame (in the pod)

1,400-calorie plan: 1 cup boiled edamame (in the pod)

1,600-calorie plan: Smoothie: 8 ounces low-fat soy milk blended with 1 cup frozen whole strawberries

1,800-calorie plan: Smoothie: 8 ounces low-fat soy milk blended with 1 cup frozen whole strawberries + ½ cup fresh blueberries or ½ banana

2,000-calorie plan: Smoothie: 8 ounces low-fat soy milk blended with 1 cup frozen whole strawberries + ½ cup fresh blueberries or ½ banana + 24 baby carrots

DINNER

Vegetable and White Bean Salad (page 179)

FUN FOOD
*Chocolate Chip Meringues (substitute carob chips for the chocolate chips) (page 277)

Day 6

BREAKFAST
*Strawberry Oat Pancakes (page 75)

LUNCH
Red Lentil Dip with Crudités and Pita Wedges (page 107)

SNACK
1,200-calorie plan: 1 rice cake topped with 1 slice soy cheese and tomato
1,400-calorie plan: 1 rice cake topped with 1 slice soy cheese and tomato
1,600-calorie plan: 1 rice cake topped with 1 slice soy cheese and tomato + ½ grapefruit, 1
    orange, 1 peach, or ¼ cantaloupe
1,800-calorie plan: 2 rice cakes topped with 1 slice soy cheese and tomato + ½ grapefruit, 1
    orange, 1 peach, or ¼ cantaloupe
2,000-calorie plan: 3 rice cakes topped with 3 slices soy cheese and tomato

DINNER
Portobello Parmesan with Broccoli Rabe (page 234)

FUN FOOD
Chunky Applesauce Pie (page 272)

Day 7

BREAKFAST
*Vegetable Frittata (page 81)

LUNCH
Grilled Vegetable Sandwich (page 115)

SNACK

1,200-calorie plan: Apple

1,400-calorie plan: Apple

1,600-calorie plan: Apple + 2 level teaspoons peanut butter

1,800-calorie plan: Apple + 1 level tablespoon peanut butter

2,000-calorie plan: Peach or orange + apple + 1 level tablespoon peanut butter

DINNER

Angel Hair Pasta Piccata (page 171)

FUN FOOD

2 Fruity Marshmallow Bars (page 261)

Index

About the Authors

Joy Bauer, M.S., R.D., C.D.N.

Joy Bauer has built one of the largest nutrition centers in the country. Located in Manhattan and Westchester, Joy Bauer Nutrition provides counseling to both adults and children dealing with a variety of nutritional concerns, including weight management, diabetes, eating disorders, cardiac rehabilitation, sports nutrition, food allergies, gastrointestinal disorders, pregnancy, lactation, and menopause.

Recognized as one of the leading nutrition authorities, Joy has a clientele that includes high-profile professionals, celebrity actors, fashion models, and Olympic athletes. She regularly appears on television shows, including *Today in New York*, *The View*, and VH1, and is continuously interviewed and featured in national publications, including *Self*, *In Touch*, *Cosmopolitan*, *Marie Claire*, *Harper's Bazaar*, *Vogue*, *Glamour*, *US Weekly*, *Ladies' Home Journal*, *Family Circle*, *Men's Fitness*, *Woman's Day*, *Allure*, *Seventeen*, *Parenting*, *Cosmo Girl*, *Teen People*, and *The New York Daily News*. In addition, Joy is a contributing editor and has a monthly column in *Self* magazine and regularly lectures and conducts workshops on nutrition and fitness across the United States.

Joy is the author of *The Complete Idiot's Guide to Total Nutrition*, and *The 90/10 Weight-Loss Plan*, both bestsellers.

Joy received her bachelor's degree in Kinesiological Sciences from the University of Maryland and a master's of science in nutrition from New York University. In the beginning of her career, Joy completed a five-year post as Director of Nutrition and Fitness for the "Heart-Smart Kids Program"—a program that she developed for the Mount Sinai Medical Center's Department of Pediatric Cardiology in New York City. Joy also served as nutrition consultant to the Columbia Presbyterian Medical Center, where she designed and supervised their ongoing research in eating disorders and weight management. Furthermore, Joy served as the clinical nutritionist with the

Neurosurgical team at Mount Sinai Medical Center and taught anatomy and physiology and sports nutrition at New York University's School of Continuing and Professional Studies. She was also the exclusive nutritionist for New York University's faculty, students, and athletes.

Joy lives in New York with her husband, Ian; her daughters, Jesse and Ayden Jane; and her son Cole. Joy's Web site is www.joybauernutrition.com.

Rosemary Black

Rosemary Black, food editor of the New York *Daily News,* is a frequent contributor to *Parenting, Ladies' Home Journal, American Baby,* and *Family Circle.* She is the author of *The Kids' Holiday Baking Book.* Rosemary lives with her husband and six children in Westchester County, New York.